AMERICAN FEDERALISM IN PRACTICE

AMERICAN FEDERALISM IN PRACTICE

THE FORMULATION AND IMPLEMENTATION OF CONTEMPORARY HEALTH POLICY

MICHAEL DOONAN

BROOKINGS INSTITUTION PRESS
Washington, D.C.

Copyright © 2013
THE BROOKINGS INSTITUTION
1775 Massachusetts Avenue, N.W., Washington, DC 20036
www.brookings.edu

Library of Congress Cataloging-in-Publication data
Doonan, Michael (Michael T.)
  American federalism in practice : the formulation and implementation of con-temporary health policy / Michael Doonan.
    pages   cm
  Includes bibliographical references and index.
  ISBN 978-0-8157-2483-4 (pbk. : alk. paper)
  1. State Children's Health Insurance Program (U.S.) 2. United States. Health Insurance Portability and Accountability Act of 1996. 3. Health insurance—United States. 4. Health insurance—Massachusetts. 5. Child health services—United States. 6. Child health services—Massachusetts. I. Title.
  RJ102.D66 2013
  368.38'20083—dc23   2013022073

9 8 7 6 5 4 3 2 1

Printed on acid-free paper

Typeset in Minion

Composition by Cynthia Stock
Silver Spring, Maryland

Printed by R. R. Donnelley
Harrisonburg, Virginia

CONTENTS

ACKNOWLEDGMENTS

This book is the result of more than a decade of exploration of intergovernmental relations and U.S. health care reform at the national and state levels. It has been influenced by my work in Congress, for federal government agencies, and with the states as well as by my academic work at the Heller School for Social Policy and Management at Brandeis University, the Politics Department at Brandeis, and the George Washington University. It is informed by a wide range of practitioners and academics who gave freely of their time, knowledge, and insight.

The idea of studying federalism across the policy process came from discussions with and reviews by Jeff Prottas, Deborah Stone, and John McDonough, and this study has been influenced by the thinking of each of these individuals. My understanding of the historical roots of federalism within the broader institutional framework benefited from the guidance of Sid Milkis; notions of the trade-off between accountability and reliability came from a course that I took with Shep Melnick. The theories of federalism that underpin this work are based on seminal studies by Daniel Elazar, Samuel Beer, Martha Derthick, Timothy Conlan, Paul Peterson, and many others.

Insight into Massachusetts reform came from Phil Johnston and Sarah Iselin and from the work on Massachusetts health care reform by the Blue Cross Blue Shield of Massachusetts Foundation. The wisdom and mentorship of Stuart Altman has enriched this study and kept me on track. David Shactman provided critical insight and support on many of the chapters. Brian Rosman reviewed the Massachusetts chapter in detail, and James Morone and Dan Ehlke reviewed a chapter on Massachusetts reform that they included in their commendable textbook, *Health Politics and Policy*.

Much of the data and information on the cases came from senior congressional staff on both sides of the aisle; White House officials; senior state officials; representatives of state organizations such as the National Governors Association, the National Conference of State Legislatures, and the National Association of Insurance Commissions; and public interest groups such as the Children's Defense Fund, Child Welfare League, Health Care for All of Massachusetts, and others. Many are cited; others provided politically sensitive information not for direct attribution. The intellect, dedication, and tireless efforts of these officials eviscerate stereotypes of disengaged "bureaucrats" and reinforce the notion of honorable public service.

Lisa Lynch, the dean of the Heller School, provided support, advice, and sabbatical coverage, all of which were essential to this work and are much appreciated. Research support and editing were provided by Jaclyn Rappaport, Nicole Hudson, Kate Tull, Susan Houghton, Erin Doonan, and Chris Woolston. Every day I am energized by my students in the Master's of Public Policy Program at the Heller School and bolstered by colleagues Janet Bogaslaw, Norma DeMattos, Mary Brolin, Corinne Kyriacou, Shelly Steenrod, and Sarah Rudy. Special thanks to Chris Kelaher from the Brookings Institution Press for his confidence in this project, guidance, and professionalism. Brookings Press editor Eileen Hughes made significant contributions that pushed the book over the finish line.

The book is dedicated to my parents, J. Peter and Dolores Doonan, whose encouragement and support know no bounds and whose multiple reviews added clarity. My partner Patty and daughters Samantha and Chloe make it all worthwhile.

CHAPTER ONE

FEDERALISM
CREATES HEALTH
POLICY

Friends in my small town know that I have been involved in national health care reform efforts as well as those in our home state of Massachusetts. When conversation at the local pub turns to health care, they'll ask me questions. Because I'm a political scientist, not a medical doctor, I don't get pelted with questions everywhere I go, so I welcome the opportunity to respond. I only wish that there were better answers.

Jack, a salesman for a high-tech company, thought that the Massachusetts health care reform would allow him to cover his 24-year-old daughter, Meghan, on his employer's health plan. So why did his company tell him that she wasn't covered? I try to explain that larger companies are exempt from state insurance regulations because they self-insure; those businesses use insurance companies like Blue Cross or Aetna only to administer their claims. It is confusing because the same insurance companies actually provide insurance to small businesses, and in those cases they are subject to state regulations. Eyes glaze over, and we quickly return to the fortunes of the Boston Red Sox. Meanwhile, Meghan remained uninsured.

Matthew runs a small financial consulting business. Because of double-digit health insurance premium increases, coverage for him, his wife, and their three boys takes a big bite out of their budget. He wanted to know whether health care reform would offer more reasonably priced health plans. A while back, I had told him that help was on the way: Massachusetts had just created the Health Care Connector, which was intended to provide a choice of plans at lower prices, at least in theory. The Connector did expand coverage to lower-income individuals and families, but it did not lower the cost of insurance for people like Matt and his family. Perhaps I should have told him to hold tight for federal small business tax credits? Or let him know that health care exchanges created by national reform may offer a better solution soon? But at the risk of losing credibility and a good tennis partner, I turn back to discussing the ball game.

As the country geared up for national health care reform, I traveled from state to state talking about reform efforts in Massachusetts. Everywhere I went, I shared my excitement over the obvious progress in coverage. More than 98 percent of people in Massachusetts have health insurance, by far the highest coverage rate in the nation. Enacted in 2006, state reform added a patchwork of new programs and regulations that built on previous expansion efforts. Over 300,000 previously uninsured individuals now have health insurance coverage and can sleep better at night. But the program is complex and difficult to comprehend—even for policy wonks—and it was not designed to address persistently rising health care costs.

National health care reform was signed into law by President Obama on March 23, 2010. The Patient Protection and Affordable Care Act (ACA) has much in common with the Massachusetts effort. It holds similar promise— and suffers from similar limitations—when it comes to expanding health care coverage to the uninsured. More of the uninsured will be covered, but coverage will be complex to negotiate and cost containment will be just as difficult. Despite its shortcomings, ACA represents a significant political triumph after a series of failed efforts that date back to the Truman administration.[1] Under national guidelines, reform will be administered in large part by the states through existing health plans, insurers, hospitals, doctors, and other health care providers.[2] States will be critical players in implementing reform and in establishing state-based health care exchanges. Applying national exchange rules to health systems that vary widely from state to state will be a tremendous challenge.

The ACA barely passed Congress, along partisan lines. The Democrats struggled to hold on to more conservative members of their party and used parliamentary maneuvers to avert defeat by filibuster in the Senate. The Democrats in the Senate did not even have the votes to include a relatively modest "public option" insurance plan to help balance private sector offerings and force down administrative costs. However, it is unlikely that anything more progressive could have passed. In fact, after the 2010 election, when the Republicans gained control of the House of Representatives and the conservative Tea Party adherents attacked the ACA as the centerpiece of their "revolution," the Democrats were fighting repeal.

Universal or near universal coverage has been referred to as the unfinished business of the New Deal. The New Deal represented a major realignment of the political parties in favor of social welfare policy, and efforts to improve, modify, and build on it have been a subject of political debate for decades.[3] In this case, the advantage went to the Democrats. The election of Ronald Reagan in the 1980s represented a realignment against social welfare policy expansion and the national agenda of the Great Society and War on Poverty programs of the 1960s and 1970s. In the 1990s, Speaker of the House Newt Gingrich took the Reagan revolution one step further, taking aim at the New Deal with efforts to privatize portions of Social Security and Medicare.[4] In this case, the Republicans had the advantage. Today the proper role of government and its role in health care reform is still hotly debated. The success or failure of the implementation of the ACA may well determine which political party holds sway over the next several decades.

Conservative opposition to the ACA represented not only an attack on a particular piece of legislation but an ongoing fight about the legitimacy of the government's efforts to ensure health care security for citizens. While repeal passed the House several times in 2012, the Democrats, who controlled the Senate, protected the law. Even if the Senate were controlled by the Republicans, it would still take sixty votes even to end the debate and have a vote on repeal. The American political system is structured to make passing legislation hard, which makes passing repeal equally challenging.

The ACA also dodged two near-death experiences. The first was the Supreme Court decision in *National Federation of Independent Business (NFIB) v. Sebelius,* which found the individual mandate requiring people to purchase health insurance to be constitutional.[5] Without the mandate, much of the ACA falls apart. The law prevents insurance companies from denying coverage for people with preexisting conditions and requires them to make products widely available and renewable in their service area. Without a coverage mandate, people could simply wait until they got sick or needed care to sign up for insurance and then drop coverage when they were well. Doing that flies in the face of the concept of insurance. Furthermore, implementing the ACA without the mandate would lead to lower numbers of younger, healthier people enrolling in the health exchanges, leaving disproportionately older and sicker people in what insurers call the risk pool. That would increase costs and make insurance even less attractive to healthier people, creating still higher costs and an insurance death spiral. Finally, the mandate is essential to covering the 30 million uninsured people that the law is designed to cover.

The second bullet was dodged with the reelection of President Obama. His challenger, Mitt Romney, vowed to begin the repeal process through executive orders on his first day in office. A Romney win would have empowered and emboldened opponents of reform in Congress and in state houses throughout the country. Furthermore, a large number of states were sitting on the fence, awaiting the election results before moving forward in earnest with implementation.[6] In addition, a Romney administration could have significantly weakened the ACA through the administrative rulemaking process. Nevertheless, the Court ruling and the election merely kept reform alive; the political battle continues through the rulemaking process and state implementation.

Making the ACA a reality will be a complex process fraught with peril. How enthusiastic will the twenty-seven states that were part of the lawsuit against reform be about implementing the major provisions of the law? Further significant opposition continues in Congress, and public opinion on reform is split. In particular, 60 percent of the population is opposed to the individual mandate.[7] The political right still characterizes the ACA as "socialized medicine" and a "massive government takeover of the health care system." Certainly it represents an expansion of government intervention, but health plans, insurers, hospitals, and physicians and other providers all remain private or not-for-profit entities. Missteps in implementation will reinforce notions of government incompetence and increase calls for greater privatization. The political and individual stakes are high.

Success would be hard to reverse. Once the policy is in place, a powerful political coalition is likely to develop to protect gains. The program has the potential to enjoy the kind of broad political support enjoyed by Medicare, Social Security, and unemployment insurance. If the plan succeeds in covering 30 million additional Americans, who will be clamoring for the "good old days" when millions could not pay their hospital bills and people were denied coverage for preexisting conditions? Ultimately, the fate of reform rests on implementation and on intergovernmental relations within the framework of American federalism. The states are at the epicenter of implementation, and their actions will be guided by federal rules and regulations.[8] The interplay between the states and the federal government will determine, for example, how the new health care exchanges will vary between states. It will also dictate the following:

—how federal tax-based subsidies will be administered through state-based health exchanges

—how new insurance regulations will dovetail with existing state laws and systems

—how states can use the new flexibility to alter the benefits for Medicaid beneficiaries

—whether states agree to expand Medicaid to all low-income individuals and families with an income below 133 percent of the federal poverty level

—how the individual mandate for insurance coverage will be enforced

—who will determine what is considered "affordable" for the purpose of enforcing the mandate

—who will set and enforce minimal benefit standards

—how sanctions on individuals and business will be administered.

In short, intergovernmental relations will shape the program and determine whether reform will reach its coverage and cost-containment goals.

If I tried to explain the importance of federalism and intergovernmental relations to Jack and Matt, not only would their eyes glaze over, but the guys would probably get up and leave me at the bar. Yet federal-state interactions determine the success or failure of policy and programs that impact us all. Knowledge about intergovernmental relations is essential to understand the policy process, to evaluate options for effective and politically feasible implementation, and to understand how programs operate. Such insight, which can be obtained only by systematically examining intergovernmental relations for different types of policy across the policy process, is essential for scholars and students of public policy as well as practitioners at the national, state, and local level who struggle to make programs work.

A more comprehensive understanding of American federalism in practice and its impact on programs and policy comes from three case studies—the State Children's Health Insurance Program (CHIP), the Health Insurance Portability and Accountability Act (HIPAA), and the health care reform enacted by Massachusetts. Each mirrors key elements of the ACA and offers unique insights into policy formulation and implementation. CHIP is an example of coverage expansion, with state flexibility and federal oversight. HIPAA is an example of insurance regulation, with federal standards but limited national resources and weak oversight of state activity. The Massachusetts reform has many similarities to national reform, but within a policy environment that is significantly different from that of the majority of states. Each case demonstrates that states can be a source of innovation for social welfare policy, particularly during times of national policy gridlock. Each case provides lessons in how the ACA might be successfully—or unsuccessfully—implemented.

The book is divided into three sections, each of which addresses one of the three case studies. Within the sections are chapters on federal-state relations as they apply to legislative development, rulemaking, and implementation. The final chapter draws conclusions from all the cases regarding how federalism affects both program development and the policy process and applies what has been learned to the implementation of national health care reform.

CHIP, HIPAA, AND MASSACHUSETTS REFORM

CHIP, passed in 1997, provides grants to the states to expand health insurance coverage to uninsured children whose family income is too high to qualify for Medicaid but who lack access to private insurance. The program has been an enormously successful federal-state partnership resulting in health insurance for millions of uninsured children. In 2010, the program covered more than 7 million children. National reform in 2010 extended CHIP until 2019 and provided supplemental federal funding, along with a requirement that states continue to maintain coverage levels.

As with many policies, a good deal of work occurred before most of the federal rules relating to CHIP were put in place and details ironed out. States were encouraged to innovate by designing alternative programs, and they received incentives to participate through increased federal reimbursements. State implementation was kept in line through significant federal oversight and mandatory reporting requirements. From the outset, CHIP provided states with the flexibility to design their own program or expand Medicaid or to come up with some combination of those two options. Within federal guidelines, states could set eligibility rules, benefit levels, provider payments, and other program requirements. The result was not only a major expansion of coverage but also great equalization in coverage levels across states.

HIPAA, which passed in 1996, had a host of goals, including privacy protection, regulation of insurance, prevention of fraud and abuse, simplification of administrative tasks, and creation of medical savings accounts. The focus here is on the portion of the HIPAA that addresses insurance regulation, including limiting exclusions for preexisting conditions and guaranteeing policy renewal. These aims are similar to those of national insurance reform in the ACA. HIPAA standards were meant to extend federal control in an area traditionally regulated by the states, but unlike with CHIP, federal resources, administrative expertise, and oversight were so limited that states largely controlled the process nevertheless. Ultimately, there remained wide variation between states and the regulations had limited impact, hence the need for significant insurance regulation in the ACA.

The third case, Massachusetts health care reform, served as a model for national reform, even if presidential candidate and former Massachusetts governor Mitt Romney later denied it. Both plans include an individual mandate to purchase insurance, health care purchasing exchanges, expansion of the Medicaid program, and subsidies for low- and moderate-income individuals and families. The reform was based on the notion of shared responsibility, and Massachusetts asked individuals, businesses, and government to

pitch in. Individuals must purchase health insurance if it is deemed affordable, or they face a fine. Businesses with eleven or more full-time employees
must provide health insurance or pay a small fee. In order to increase affordability, the state government, with federal support, expanded subsidies to
low- and moderate-income residents.

From the beginning, Massachusetts reform depended on support from
the federal government. Through a federal government Medicaid waiver, the
state was receiving millions of dollars paid directly to hospitals for uncompensated care. The George W. Bush administration threatened to stop providing this money, $385 million a year, if the state did not shift funding
away from hospitals and toward direct coverage of the uninsured. Interest-
ingly, the conservative Bush administration pushed for reform and approved
the plan that would ultimately serve as a model for "Obamacare," which is
detested by the political right.

The rules for determining exactly how Massachusetts reform would work
were developed in large part by the Commonwealth Health Care Connector
Authority Board, which is made up of representatives from government,
business, labor, and consumer organizations. With significant autonomy,
the board sets benefit and subsidy levels and determines what is considered
affordable insurance at particular income levels. Rules for other components
of reform, such as Medicaid expansion, tax policy, and business and labor
regulations, were written by the appropriate state agencies in collaboration
with the Connector board. Under tight deadlines, the job got done, with
both the state and the federal government watching every step.

AMERICAN FEDERALISM

Understanding how federalism—the division of power between the federal
government and the states—plays out is essential to understanding contemporary health policy. The case studies presented here describe a dynamic
intergovernmental relationship that varies dramatically depending on the
political context in each case and the manner within each state in which
rulemaking and implementation are conducted. Health policymaking is
entangled in a complex web of shared, overlapping, and/or competing power
relationships between levels of government.[9] While traditional studies of
federalism offer great insight into federal-state interactions, most do little to
explain variations in interactions across the policy process. Understanding
those variations is essential to understanding the ultimate impact of federalism on programs and policy.

Traditionally, particular models of federalism were ascribed to specific historical periods.[10] Prior to the New Deal in the 1930s, most domestic responsibilities in the United States were handled in the realms of state and local governments, charities, and families. Under the New Deal, the federal government worked with states to address poverty and unemployment, expanding the role of government and building administrative capacity at the national and state levels in the process. States remained active partners, in part because powerful Southern members of Congress fought for control of federal aid to prevent it from benefiting African Americans.[11] After victory in World War II and the onset of the cold war, international attention turned to Washington, D.C. Domestically, the postwar period was one of unprecedented economic growth, and people looked increasingly to the national government for services and support. The difference in professionalism between the national and state governments was stark. Around the time that President Kennedy promised to send a man to the moon, the evening news showed a governor blocking African American children from going to school and state police turning fire hoses on peaceful civil rights marchers.

In the 1960s, in contrast to the states, the federal government declared war on poverty and pledged to create a "Great Society" focused on promoting human development, civil rights, the arts, and environmental protection.[12] Under President Lyndon Johnson, efforts to attain those goals expanded the reach of the federal government to every corner of the nation. The federal government often bypassed the states to work with and empower local communities through initiatives such as Head Start, community development block grants, community health centers, and legal aid.

However, that hard-won public trust in the federal government soon waned. The Vietnam War, the resignation of President Nixon, rampant inflation, the Iran hostage crisis, and renewed racial tension and urban unrest weakened the standing and credibility of the national government. Confidence in Washington and its ability to address social problems diminished.

Ronald Reagan's presidency, in the 1980s, is considered a period of devolution of power from the federal government to the states. Reagan famously stated, "Government is not the solution to our problems; government is the problem," and that message resonated with many Americans. Taxes were reduced, and government programs were cut or curtailed. The brakes were put on innovation in national social welfare policy. The period also saw a rash of unfunded mandates placed on the states, particularly in the Medicaid program.[13] Ever-mounting deficits and the national debt further restricted national domestic policy initiatives.

Within that larger framework, much of the research on federalism involving health policy focused on finding a grand theory to describe federal-state relations during a particular period of time.[14] After Bill Clinton failed to enact health care reform, Robert Rich and William White concluded in their 1996 volume, *Health Policy, Federalism, and the American States,* that "we are on the threshold of a new era of federalism in health care . . . decisions made in the next several years may set the course of federalism in health care and other major social policy areas well into the next century."[15] Some studies described federalism as a pendulum swinging between state and federal dominance.[16] Others explored theories about which models of federalism were most effective in implementing certain types of programs. Paul Peterson grouped policies into distributive, redistributive, and developmental categories, theorizing that certain programs are most effectively implemented under particular models.[17] Other researchers made a case for a certain type of federal relationship that they believed to be spelled out in the Constitution.[18] Most studies focused on the legislative process and neglected rulemaking and implementation.

As a member of President Clinton's health care task force and later as a fellow for the Senate Finance Committee, I witnessed that round of health care reform fail in a spectacular fashion. Discouraged, I left government, returned to academia and took up Rich and White's challenge of finding a new model of federalism that would describe federal-state relations. The goal was to get ready for the next round of reform; with diminished opportunity for national reform, I focused on the states and intergovernmental relations.

The problem was that no single model was useful in clarifying how and why federalism plays out in particular ways for specific programs. For example, one overarching theory of federalism helps in understanding the contrast between the growth of the federal government in the 1960s and its lack of growth in other eras, such as the 1980s, when attempts were made to reduce its reach. However, it does very little to explain the completely different intergovernmental relationships pertaining to Medicare (federal health insurance for people over 65 years of age) and Medicaid (health insurance for low-income families administered by the states with federal matching funds), which were passed at the same time.[19] Macro federalism theory does little to explain why, for example, Medicare Part D (which provides prescription drug coverage to seniors) significantly expanded federal government power and spending at a time when conservatives controlled the White House and Congress, an era when power was supposedly leaving Washington and returning to the states.

Understanding how power and authority determine winners and losers in public policy requires building on existing theory and drilling deeper into the policymaking process. It requires more detailed program- and policy-level analysis within the broader context of the American political system. It requires close-up examination of rulemaking and implementation. Peterson, Rabe, and Wong's *When Federalism Works* provides such an analysis of federalism at the program level, with a focus on implementation within the broader political context.[20] The journal *Publius* also publishes annual assessments of federalism under various administrations.[21] The analysis that I present in this volume uses policy and programs as the unit of analysis and shows that increasingly, federalism goals are subservient to political ambitions. This volume also is inspired by the work of a long line of federalism scholars, particularly Timothy Conlan, who says, "Today the design, operation, and performance of most federal domestic programs cannot be understood without an intergovernmental perspective."[22] His analysis, which proves that statement to be true, is a springboard for this work.

Building on past theoretical and empirical work, I track intergovernmental relations across the policy process for each of three case studies, which are based on data and evidence that I collected from detailed interviews with federal and state officials, legislators, and staff and consumer and interest group leaders. I also analyze primary and secondary documents—including legislative language, records of hearings and testimony, administrative rules included in the *Federal Register,* and a range of documents concerning implementation. This systematic approach will help in better understanding how federalism shapes policy and affects people.

THE POLICY PROCESS

For the purpose of this analysis, federalism needs to be studied across the policy process, including not only how legislation is crafted but also how administrative rules are written and policies and programs are implemented.

The Legislature

The structure of federal-state relations with respect to any policy begins with the legislative process. For example, the way that Congress structured health exchanges in the ACA set up federal-state relations in a way that has particular policy implications. The law establishes exchanges as state-based organizations through which individuals and small groups can select from a range of health plans. But it did not have to be that way. After rejecting a national public option health plan, Congress chose the Senate plan for state-based exchanges instead of the House plan for a national health insurance exchange. A national exchange would have maximized federal power to regulate health insurance offerings, creating more uniformity, but reduced state variation and flexibility. State-based exchanges require the federal government and the states to share power and authority. As a result, more variation will occur across state insurance exchanges. Down the road, when health exchanges provide radically different services in Texas and Minnesota, for example, that critical decision will help explain why.

Although more liberal members of Congress were pushing for national exchanges, it is not always the case that conservatives support states' rights and liberals support increased federal authority. Timothy Conlan demonstrates a direct link between a policymaker's position on federalism and policy preferences in his examination of federalism and the policy and program agendas of presidents Nixon and Reagan and Speaker of the House Newt Gingrich.[23] In fact, conservatives have often supported national uniformity to protect their interests, such as national standards to limit abortion services, same sex marriages, and business regulation. For example, during the CHIP reauthorization in 2008, George W. Bush supported national standards in order to deny states the option of providing health insurance to parents of CHIP-covered children and to uninsured middle-class children.

Conversely, liberals support greater state rights when it aligns with their interests, such as stronger consumer protections or increased coverage for abortions. In the case of HIPAA, the late liberal senator Paul Wellstone (D-Minn.) made the strongest pitch that states should have the flexibility to provide health insurance–related consumer protections that exceed federal minimums if they choose. In 2012, Representative Barney Frank (D-Mass.) supported states' right to legislate same-sex marriage laws.[24] The findings here support the claim that when ideals about federalism clash with interests, interests win.

Rulemaking

Politics does not end when legislation is passed; it continues into the rulemaking and implementation phases. In making policy, the importance of the rules and regulations developed by the executive branch almost rival the importance of the originating legislation. Although it has recently received more attention, rulemaking has often been neglected in the study of public policy.[25] Federal rulemaking is a relatively open process, crafted with input from various stakeholders, including the states. It is more open to interest groups that have the legal and technical resources to follow complex undertakings and far less open to the general public, which has relatively more input into the legislative process.[26] Draft rules are regularly published in the *Federal Register*, with a specified comment period. In the case of health insurance exchanges, the Department of Health and Human Services, in cooperation with other federal agencies, will define operational methods, eligibility for subsidies, minimum benefit levels, maximum out-of-pocket costs, and regulation of premiums. The rule will define the degree to which each level of government sets, defines, and enforces standards. As these critical decisions are made, interest groups have another chance to advance policies that they favor and block or weaken regulations that they oppose. One could imagine that hospitals, physicians, other providers, consumer groups, business, consumer advocacy organizations and various subgroups of these organizations would be very interested in influencing how critical policy questions are answered. Studying the rulemaking process is essential to understanding federalism and the locus of power and authority to make critical program and policy decisions.

Implementation

Once the rules are crafted, it is up to the states, federal government, and stakeholder organizations to implement policy. The American political system has a long-standing bias against government in general and against a strong federal bureaucracy in particular. The case is rarely made for a powerful national bureaucracy, except during wartime. The states, not-for-profit organizations, and the private sector are looked to for implementation. This is true even for the national Medicare program: private physicians and for-profit and not-for-profit hospitals provide the services; fiscal intermediaries are hired to evaluate claims and pay the bills.[27] Even contemporary Democratic leaders are against "bureaucracy." President Bill Clinton declared that "the era of big government is over," and President Barack Obama campaigned not to make government "bigger" but to make it "smarter." There is little support in the United States for a one-size-fits-all policy handed down by Washington. As a consequence, arguments supporting federal action are generally indirect, ignoring issues of federalism and instead supporting notions such as "fiscal prudence," "family values," or "private sector job growth." Again, it is important to look behind federalism rhetoric for particular interests.

The law and the rules guide implementation, but the cases presented here make clear that program resources, sanctions, administrative capacity, and reporting requirements and the enthusiasm or support for a policy or program also are important. Historically, it has been difficult to get sovereign states with independent power to faithfully implement policy that they find objectionable. For example, the constitutionally protected civil rights of former slaves, enacted after the Civil War during Reconstruction, dissolved when federal troops left the South. Much later, court-ordered integration of public schools suffered from lack of effective implementation. In each case, limited federal sanctions, oversight, and resources combined with powerful state and local opposition to thwart national policy. However, strong federal parameters, along with carrots and sticks, could lead states to implement reform that significantly expands access to quality health insurance across the country. Findings from the CHIP case study indicate that state flexibility constrained by federal guidelines can expand access to comprehensive health insurance coverage and allow state innovation in how the health care delivery system is structured. As stated previously, CHIP was well financed and had strong federal reporting requirements and oversight—characteristics that led to a significant degree of uniformity and a high level of health insurance coverage for children across the states. That suggests that the considerable federal funding included in the ACA to expand Medicaid could have similar success, but it is not guaranteed. HIPAA, on the other hand, had weak federal oversight, limited reporting requirements, and insignificant state funding. In part, those deficiencies led to a mix of outcomes across the country and to questionable impact.

Intergovernmental relationships are far from set with the passage of legislation. Structuring these relationships remains a tool during rulemaking and implementation, when interests can attempt to strengthen, weaken, or solidify gains made during the legislative process.

The dance of intergovernmental relations within the federal system is a critical part of policy innovation in the United States. CHIP demonstrated that what began as modest state efforts to expand health insurance coverage for children could lead to a bipartisan effort in Congress to cover millions of children nationwide. The Massachusetts reform demonstrated that significant federal funding and cooperation were necessary for the state effort to move toward universal coverage. CHIP and Massachusetts reform were bipartisan efforts that leveraged considerable federal funding. Both cases suggest that state action is a helpful and possibly a necessary precursor to the enactment of progressive health policy. Richard Nathan refers to such state action as "liberals discovering federalism."[28] Each case, HIPAA in particular, highlights the importance of resources, funding, administrative capacity, and intergovernmental coordination for achieving program success.

Implications for National Reform

Lessons from the case studies offer insight into how health policy is constructed and implemented and how it can be applied to the current round of national reform. As with CHIP, the successful implementation of national reform requires a balance between state flexibility and national accountability. Federal command-and-control regulations will not work, partly because state health care systems are so diverse. Furthermore, states have the political power to resist, either by raising public opposition or by dragging their feet. Alternatively, ceding too much control to the states can lead to wide disparities in achievement of coverage and cost containment goals and increases the danger that funds will be inappropriately spent.

Finding the correct balance is the real challenge. The federal government must have the capacity to compel state action and the ability and willingness to work collaboratively with states to apply rules to their unique health care systems. The federal government can strengthen its authority by tying federal money to state compliance, issuing mandatory reporting requirements, and being able and willing to take corrective action. States can increase their power by taking full advantage of their administrative capacity and expertise. Furthermore, the process of state implementation confers its own flexibility, as federal officials are kept at arm's length. There also needs to be congruence between the goals of the program and the historical mission of the responsible federal agency. That may mean that different aspects of reform are implemented by different federal agencies. For example, the Centers for Medicare and Medicaid Services (CMS) is responsible for working with states on Medicaid expansion. CMS has expertise, established relationships, and a pot of gold to encourage state cooperation, so programmatically, Medicaid expansion should be relatively straightforward.

Setting up national health care exchanges will be a far more challenging task. Again, CMS is charged with taking the lead in writing the regulations and overseeing state implementation. However, this task is not a core element of the agency's historical mission, and it does not have preexisting expertise or routines. Because each state has a unique set of insurance regulations and its own mix of public and private health care insurance options, the task will be difficult, and collaboration will be needed if the effort is to succeed. The federal government should be prepared to work with states more as a partner and less as a regulator. But allowing too much leeway could lead to the same kind of failures that occurred with HIPAA.

The Massachusetts case is both comforting and scary. It demonstrates that the individual mandate is essential to institute insurance market reforms and achieve coverage expansion. Fears that employers in Massachusetts would drop coverage and push people into the state exchange were not realized. In addition, the plan did not increase per capita costs in the state relative to those in the rest of the nation, as some had predicted. Massachusetts reform was successful in large part because it was bipartisan and stakeholders were engaged and supportive, especially during implementation. While President Obama did a much better job of engaging stakeholders than Bill Clinton did, his plan was passed along purely partisan lines, and that fact will make implementation difficult. Furthermore, Massachusetts showed that the individual mandate will not be self-implementing. It will take significant outreach on the statewide and community level.

Politics is ongoing during rulemaking and implementation. With national reform, the left or right may try to use "maximum state flexibility" to weaken provisions of a bill that they oppose. The right may seek to limit potential adverse effects on business and reduce the overall scope and cost of the law. The left may seek to provide more state flexibility to cover abortion services or permit implementation of a state-based single-payer system. Opponents of national reform have already said that they intend to reduce funding for implementation, threatening to prevent the Internal Revenue Service from carrying out its responsibility to enforce the individual mandate. What should be clear is that understanding federalism and politics at each level of the policymaking process is critical to recognizing where and how critical policy decisions are made and carried out.

CHAPTER TWO

CHIP:
FEDERALISM
IN CONGRESS

The State Children's Health Insurance Program of 1997 (CHIP) was enacted during an especially turbulent time in American politics. The Clinton health care plan had failed, and conservative members of Congress were emboldened to make some big moves. Under the leadership of Speaker of the House Newt Gingrich, Republicans passed a plan to end the federal entitlement to Medicaid and replace it with block grants to the states. In a showdown with Congress, President Clinton vetoed the bill, shut down the government, and eventually saved the program. Incredibly, that was the environment that gave birth to what was at the time the largest health insurance coverage expansion since Medicare and Medicaid in the 1960s.

The history of CHIP illustrates how the balance of power between the states and the federal government shapes health policy. Issues of federalism were critical in the passage of the program. Liberal and conservative legislators both used arguments based on federalism and states' rights to forward their own policy ends. Such arguments have traditionally been used to thwart national policy. Here, they forwarded progressive national objectives.

THE BEGINNING

CHIP, which was passed as part of the Balanced Budget Act of 1997, provided $20.3 billion in funding for the first five years of the program. Ultimately the program would cover more than 11 million children and significantly reduce the number of uninsured children in the United States. CHIP provides grants to states for coverage of uninsured children in families with incomes below 200 percent of the federal poverty level; states already covering children up to that level can expand coverage further. For example, if a state already covers children up to 200 percent of the poverty level, the state can use CHIP funds to expand coverage up to 250 percent. The program, jointly financed by the federal and state governments, includes revenue from an increase in the national tobacco tax.

CHIP is not an entitlement program like Medicaid. That means that there is no guarantee that an eligible child will receive benefits. If a state spends all of its allocation, no additional federal money is available to cover additional children, no matter their eligibility. Like Medicaid, CHIP is a matching program, whereby state expenditures are partially reimbursed by the federal government. In affluent states such as Massachusetts, the federal government pays 65 percent of the program costs. In poor states such as Mississippi, the matching rate is 85 percent, which means that for every dollar that the state pays, the federal government reimburses the state 85 cents.

By contrast, the Medicaid program matching rate, which is based on state per capita income, ranged between 50 and 74 percent in 2012.[1] Strangely, the federal government pays for a greater portion of CHIP than it does for covering lower-income people under the Medicaid program. The states pushed for higher funding levels, allowing them to aggressively cover uninsured children. But in 2014 a portion of Medicaid is going to catch up, and then some. Under national reform, the federal government will initially reimburse states 100 percent of their costs to cover people newly eligible for Medicaid. That amount will gradually be lowered to 90 percent. With three different Medicaid and CHIP reimbursement levels, state and federal accountants should have strong job security.

CHIP is not just better funded than Medicaid; it also is more flexible. States can use CHIP funding to expand Medicaid coverage, develop a new state program, or use a combination of those strategies. If states choose to expand Medicaid, they have to meet all of the guidelines of this complex program. If states choose to develop their own program, they have some discretion to set eligibility levels, define benefits packages, and tailor programs based on a participant's age, geographic location, or disability status. However, CHIP also includes a number of telling federal safeguards and restrictions that illustrate the power of Washington to control state policy.

POLICY ENVIRONMENT

Before CHIP was enacted, a number of states began taking matters into their own hands. For example, Massachusetts and Vermont raised cigarette taxes and used the proceeds to expand coverage to uninsured children. New York, Pennsylvania, and Florida already had programs to enable some children to obtain state-sponsored health coverage beyond Medicaid. Even though the state programs were actually quite limited, the fact that the states were doing something ultimately undermined conservative arguments that the CHIP program was a "big government" takeover of the health care system. Those arguments and cries of "socialized medicine" had helped defeat President Clinton's earlier health care reform effort. In a similar way, Massachusetts health care reform helped pave the way for national reforms under President Obama.

After the dust settled from the defeat of national reform, in early 1997, as part of its budget proposal, the Clinton administration proposed a modest child health insurance plan with significant state flexibility. The plan expanded Medicaid outreach, permitted states to cover Medicaid children for a full year, and included a modest grant program for the states ($3.75 billion over five years). The grant program was designed to give states remarkable flexibility, reflecting Clinton's background as a governor.[2] States could establish their own criteria for eligibility, benefit levels, and guidelines for copayments, among other things. With a conservative Congress, that was the best that the administration thought it could achieve—and it was not optimistic about that.

In 1997, children's health insurance was a priority for the Democrats in both the House and the Senate, but, like the administration, they were pessimistic about its chances of success. Senate minority leader Tom Daschle (D-S.D.) held a joint press conference with House minority leader Dick Gephardt (D-Mo.) in February 1997 to implore the Republicans to add children's health insurance to the legislative agenda.[3] Early in that session, Daschle introduced modest legislation to expand coverage that included tax credits and vouchers to assist low-income and moderate-income families to provide insurance for their children. The use of such traditionally conservative approaches shows that Democrats were desperate for any type of advance.

The Republican leadership in both the House and the Senate initially opposed expansion of children's health insurance. The majority leader, Senator Trent Lott (R-Miss.), considered the effort to be "salami-slicing"—an attempt by the administration to achieve incrementally what it had failed to achieve through national reform. Senate Republicans, led by senators Bob Gramm (R-Tex.), William Roth (R-Del.), and Bill Frist (R-Tenn.), did, however, introduce a modest bill to increase state funding through the maternal and child health block grant. The bill also made it easier for states to modify their Medicaid programs and included a provision to make medical savings accounts (MSAs) available for moderate-income families.

Representative Bill Thomas (R-Calif.), the chairman of the House Ways and Means Health Subcommittee, expressed caution about moving too quickly without knowing all the facts.[4] Other Republicans on the subcommittee suggested at the April 8, 1997, hearing that many uninsured children were already receiving care through safety-net providers. Many who were also eligible for Medicaid were not enrolled. Republicans were especially concerned about the danger of "crowd out" (people dropping private coverage to join subsidized programs) and the potential adverse impact of reform on the private insurance system, which was currently providing most health coverage to children. Nevertheless, budget negotiations in mid-May of 1997 included $16 billion over five years for spending on children's health insurance.

THE RHETORIC AND REALITY OF STATE LEADERSHIP

Throughout the debate in the House and Senate, people on both sides of the issue noted programs that already were under way in the states. Opponents of children's health initiatives pointed to state activity to downplay the need for federal intervention, while proponents claimed that they were building on existing state programs and used the rhetoric of federal-state partnerships to guard against arguments that CHIP was "just another big government program."

Republicans downplayed the problem of uninsured children and exaggerated state advances in an effort to forestall federal efforts. Senator Don Nickles (R-Okla.) argued that there were fewer uninsured children than claimed. He noted that thirty-one states already had programs that provided some care for children who were not eligible for Medicaid and that a new bill should not override what the states were doing "in our zest or zeal to cover this group."[5] Representative Sam Johnson (R-Tex.) stated at a House hearing that "most states have already implemented some form of program to provide children with health insurance. Do you think we are in danger of pre-empting the states before we know what the states have done and what works best?"[6] The problem with that argument was that the states were not actually doing that much to help children not eligible for Medicaid.

Prior to CHIP, only four state programs covered more than 10,000 children.[7] One of those was CaliforniaKids, a private program supported by Blue Cross of California along with Merck Pharmaceuticals, Procter and Gamble, and the California Community Foundation. However, the program focused on prevention; it did not pay for inpatient hospital care. Michael Koch, executive director of CaliforniaKids Healthcare Foundation, proudly testified that the program covered "over 14,000 children." While that was certainly better than nothing, California had 1.87 million uninsured children at the time.[8] Moreover, at that time more than 5 million were covered by California's Medicaid program.[9] The number of children in CaliforniaKids was equal to less than 1 percent of uninsured children in the state.

Senator Bob Graham (D-Fla.) testified before the Senate Finance Committee that the Florida Healthy Kids Corporation was "a good example of the confidence we can place in states in their commitment to children and their ability to fashion appropriate programs to meet their health needs."[10] The program targets children through the schools and uses school lunch program eligibility to determine subsidy eligibility.[11] When the program began in 1997, premiums for children eligible for free lunch were $5 or $10 a month, those eligible for reduced-cost lunch paid $10 to $20, and others could join the program by paying the full price. Local governments paid 18 percent of the cost, parents paid 35 percent, and the state paid the balance.[12] The program covered 36,000 children in 1997. By comparison, 1.45 million people enrolled in Florida's Medicaid program in 1997.[13] Coverage under Florida Healthy Kids, though clearly an innovative program, was still quite modest when the state had 670,000 uninsured children at the time, representing nearly one in five children in Florida.[14] Florida Healthy Kids provided less-than-comprehensive coverage to less than 5 percent of uninsured children in the state.

New York's program was more extensive. It covered 124,000 children in 1997, or about 16 percent of the 737,800 uninsured children in the state.[15] Medicaid enrollment in 1997 was just under 3 million. Although the New York program was the most comprehensive in the country, it still left many children uncovered.

The limited scope of these state programs did not diminish their importance in the policy debate. Democrats exaggerated state activities to forward their own goals. In testimony before the Senate Finance Committee, Secretary of Health and Human Services Donna Shalala claimed, "Our proposal builds on successful efforts undertaken by a number of states."[16] Similar rhetoric from the left could be heard throughout the debate in the House and Senate. However, for the most part it was just a political ploy. Democratic leaders and strategists did not say much about state activities until after they had already developed their legislative plan.[17] The strategy worked, because it helped obtain the support of moderate and, eventually, even conservative lawmakers. In this case, liberals gained the upper hand by pointing to state activities to forward a progressive national agenda.

THE HOUSE OF REPRESENTATIVES

CHIP played out very differently in the House and Senate. Republican leaders in the House opposed increasing federal funding to cover children. When forced to do it, they opted for the block grant approach, which would have provided lump-sum payments to states and allowed them to decide how to spend the money.[18] During this period, the House leadership was talking to state governors all the time, particularly the Republican governors, who were considered an important constituency.[19] The House stuck to the $16 billion budget proposal for spending on children's health—a figure arrived at in the budget negotiations of May 1997—and opted to pass the money along to the states with few restrictions. House Democrats offered an alternative proposal to expand Medicaid, but it was defeated, largely along partisan lines (223-207).[20]

House debate centered on issues of federalism. While conservatives spoke of providing maximum flexibility to the states to meet the particular needs of communities, liberals feared that not enough money and protection were included in the block grant proposal to ensure coverage of uninsured children. Representative Jim Greenwood (R-Pa.) summed up the attitude on the right: "We need to trust our governors, we need to trust our state legislators and allow them to meet the health care needs of their children in the way that best suits their states' realities."[21] On the other side, Representative Sherrod Brown (D-Ohio) stated, "We want to make sure this money goes to insure millions of children . . . not frittered away so the governors have some kind of slush fund to plug holes in their budget."[22] Representative Patsy Mink (D-Hi.) stated, "The budget fails to guarantee coverage for children and gives excessively generous authority to states. We must set minimum standards and requirements to insure that this funding is used efficiently and effectively."[23]

As the process moved from platitudes to legislation, the conservative leadership moved away from maximum state flexibility toward a balance between states' rights and federal oversight. A senior official with the Centers for Medicare and Medicaid Services (CMS) involved in the negotiations with Congress said that when particular issues were debated, "sometimes accountability won and sometimes flexibility."[24] The House Commerce Committee's addition of Hyde Amendment language preventing the use of funds for abortion services is an example of how Republicans have restricted state flexibility in the name of a socially conservative ideology.[25] Even at the height of the so-called devolution movement, conservatives, like liberals, turned to federalism to advance their political goals.

THE SENATE

The Senate Republican leadership initially opposed any federal expansion of coverage for children but was forced to act by the legislative maneuvering of senators Edward Kennedy (D-Mass.) and Orrin Hatch (R-Utah). In 1997, after the defeat of an attempt to cover uninsured children by expanding Medicaid, Kennedy and Hatch succeeded in passing the Child Bill, a groundbreaking piece of legislation that would ultimately became CHIP. The Senate proposal and ultimately CHIP itself ended up being a compromise between Democrats and Republicans, with influence from the states, in contrast to the Patient Protection and Affordable Care Act (ACA), which was passed largely along partisan lines. The compromise was possible in part because CHIP deals with children, who are generally considered a more "deserving" group because they are dependent on adults and so cannot "choose" to be uninsured.

The states' ability to leverage their political power can be seen in their successful efforts to help defeat plans to expand Medicaid, which they opposed as inflexible and proscriptive. A proposal of Senator John Chafee (R-R.I.) and Senator Jay Rockefeller (D-W.V.) to expand Medicaid was defeated in the Senate Finance Committee on June 17, 1997, by a vote of 1–9. The Clinton White House supported the expansion, and the vote was considered a defeat for the administration.[26] Governors vigorously objected to Medicaid expansion, favoring a block grant approach instead. A member of Senator Chafee's health staff stated that the senator had "lots of discussions with various governors in which the governors were adamantly opposed to the Medicaid expansion and pushed for increased flexibility."[27] She added, "They had a tremendous influence on the debate. . . . The governors were a force to be reckoned with."[28] Democratic staff also stated that the governors had considerable influence with the Republican leadership. Senator Rockefeller said, "An amazing number of governors—governors who had never evidenced an interest in children—have been calling in the last two days."[29] Senior Democratic staff confirmed that the governors pushed hard to defeat the Medicaid expansion.

THE CHILD BILL

The Child Bill—the forerunner of CHIP, proposed by senators Kennedy and Hatch—combined an increase in the tobacco tax with expanded health insurance coverage for uninsured children. Senator Kennedy was the strategist behind the effort, and working with the conservative Senator Hatch was a critical part of his approach. For his part, Senator Hatch took grief from his colleagues and was denounced by the Republican leadership and caucus.[30] The bill, offered as an amendment to the budget bill on May 21, 1997, got off to an acrimonious start. The sponsors threatened a filibuster to force a vote that the Republican leadership wanted to avoid. Senator Kennedy deftly framed the issue: "Why can't we vote on whether the Senate stands with children or with Joe Camel and the Marlboro Man?"[31] At several points in the debate, Kennedy warned colleagues that 75 percent of the country favored this approach and that if it did not get a vote or pass, it was sure to "come back again and again."[32]

The majority leader, Senator Trent Lott, used all of his leverage, including by soliciting help from President Clinton, to defeat the amendment.[33] The president reported in the press that while he favored the concept, he thought that it would hamper passage of the budget as a whole. Senator Hatch expressed frustration, saying on the Senate floor that "I think the President and the people in the White House caved here."[34] The measure was defeated on a procedural vote of 55-45. But Kennedy and Hatch kept up the pressure for action until the Senate ultimately relented.

After negotiations within the Senate Finance committee, the Child Bill, renamed CHIP, ultimately passed, with amendments, in both chambers and was signed into law by President Clinton. During that process, Hatch and other Republicans on the Finance Committee negotiated directly with the governors while Kennedy, Rockefeller, and other Democrats on the committee worked more closely with the child interest groups.[35] The governors pushed for maximum flexibility and were especially alarmed about the possible inclusion of Early Periodic Screening, Diagnosis, and Treatment (EPSDT) Program benefits for children. EPSDT, a Medicaid benefit that requires that the widest possible range of services be available to children, would significantly reduce states' ability to pare their coverage programs or mold them to resemble programs in the private sector.[36]

Meanwhile, a massive grassroots campaign by child health advocates pushed for a comprehensive benefits package, quality assurance, and uniform national standards. Advocacy groups strongly supported retaining EPSDT requirements and benefits that resembled those in Medicaid, placing themselves in opposition to the states that wanted to pursue their own options.[37] The Finance Committee bill found middle ground. It reduced the Medicaid benefit requirements and substituted an actuarial equivalent, which would ensure comprehensive benefits but provide flexibility for plans to operate more like those in the private sector.

Several amendments to reduce state flexibility were offered by members of both parties in committee and on the Senate floor. In committee, Republicans added language restricting abortion services. On the floor, Senator Chafee and Senator Rockefeller added an amendment tightening the benefits package and adding the requirement that states offer vision and hearing benefits. Senator Chafee's key staff person said, "We wanted to hold their [states'] feet to the fire and make sure that the program money was actually going for health insurance for children."[38] Senator Paul Wellstone (D-Minn.) and Senator Pete Domenici (R-N.M.) joined together to include a mental health parity provision. Senator Domenici had argued vigorously against the Child Bill when it was first proposed, but having a close relative with mental illness, he now sought to mandate state action in an area of deep personal concern. A senior Senate Republican staff person noted said Republicans generally took a hands-off philosophy to legislative issues but that if it became "their" issue they wanted to "manage it"; they wanted to "control it."[39]

WHAT THE STATES WANTED AND WHAT THEY GOT

State influence on the development of CHIP in Congress can be seen by comparing what states asked for and what was actually included in the legislation. Representatives from the National Governors Association and the National Conference of State Legislatures were clear about what states wanted: a consistent funding stream, flexibility to design and implement their own programs, and limited federal oversight. States wanted "the ability to design a program that was state specific and could build on what the states were already doing, rather than a national Medicaid expansion for kids."[40] At their annual meeting in July 1997, state governors urged the conferees to support the block grant program structure of the House bill. In a press release, the governors stated that the bill "should complement the array of children's health programs already in place."[41] They criticized the Senate's "rigid" benefits package, declaring that "a mandated package of benefits will limit the number of children covered through the new program." The governors urged the conferees to resist passing a "one-size-fits-all law that won't fit 50 different states."[42] States were also largely opposed to the tobacco tax provision, which they saw as "stealing a source of revenue."[43]

The governors succinctly outlined their goals on July 29, 1997. They pushed for flexibility and were opposed to a straight Medicaid expansion because they were frustrated that the program was growing increasingly out of their control. Throughout the 1980s new federal requirements and spiraling health care costs had expanded the program greatly. Medicaid became the fastest-growing state budget item, second only to education in terms of total expenditures. States are required to balance their budgets, so the more that is spent on Medicaid, the less there is available for education, infrastructure, environmental protection, corrections, and other state priorities. Furthermore, it is especially difficult to cut a matching program. For example, if the state is receiving a 50 percent federal match, the federal government essentially pays for half of the program. The math dictates that because of lost federal revenue, it would take two dollars in Medicaid cuts to achieve one dollar in budget savings. When it came to CHIP, if a block grant with maximum flexibility was not available, states wanted

—to allow residents to forgo Medicaid for CHIP
—to be guaranteed full funding of the program for ten years
—to allow states that already offered expanded coverage to the majority of uninsured children to be able use CHIP money for other expenses
—to eliminate the 10 percent cap on administrative expenditures included in the bill
—to eliminate the requirement to spend money on promotion and outreach
—to be given flexibility to cover children through employer-based insurance without federal permission or waivers
—to eliminate the requirement that employer-based programs cost the same or less than those provided directly through CHIP
—to provide the option for state waivers without restrictions
—to allow family coverage without waivers from the federal government.[44]

The governors found their champions in the House of Representatives. House Republicans, led by Speaker Gingrich, worked closely with the governors, who were largely motivated by their desire to avoid a new federal program. A senior Health Care Financing Administration official who provided technical assistance to Congress during this process said that House Republicans were ideologically in camp with the states.[45] In the Senate, the governors were successful in defeating a Medicaid expansion and in loosening benefit requirements in the final package. Still, the end result was far removed from the no-strings-attached block grant that they really wanted. The Senate bill was a compromise between a block grant and a Medicaid expansion. It gave states some flexibility to develop their own programs, but it included a number of state requirements that were supported by federal legislators on the left and on the right. This is the approach that finally became law.

Chris Jennings, senior White House adviser to the president on health, described CHIP as a grand compromise: an "amalgamation of everyone's interests . . . a model of what compromise between advocacy groups, state-based interests, and Congress (Democrats and Republicans) really is." He said that the legislation found an appropriate balance "between resources, flexibility, and accountability."[46] States were successful in obtaining a significant funding stream for a guaranteed period of time. They were successful in securing the flexibility to develop their own programs. Consumer groups were successful in requiring a comprehensive benefits package and cost-sharing limitations. Congress also included a number of accountability requirements. Conservatives who were opposed to the law found it increasingly difficult to vote against coverage for children, particularly when children's coverage was pitted against big tobacco.

THE STATUTE

Analysis of the CHIP statute reveals a series of "ands," "buts," and other contingencies that guide state action while leaving room for innovation. States that chose to create their own programs had flexibility to devise plans that operated more like private sector plans and less like Medicaid. However, they still had to adhere to certain federal standards with respect to administration, eligibility, benefits, cost sharing, reporting requirements, and protections against fraud.

The benefit compromise, while allowing state plans to operate more like private sector plans, nevertheless required comprehensive benefits. Further, a number of benefits were specifically required and others explicitly prohibited. Abortion services were excluded, as were drugs to assist in suicide, euthanasia, or mercy killing.[47] The benchmark or base plan that states were required to offer had to include inpatient care, outpatient care, and a host of preventive services. There was considerable debate in conference committee over drug coverage and mental health, vision, and hearing services. The compromise agreement required that if those services are provided by the benchmark plan, at least 75 percent of the actuarial value of the services must be provided to CHIP recipients.

Similarly, states have some flexibility to determine program eligibility. Coverage is limited to children under the age of 19, and the states have to cover lower-income children before those from higher-income families. Within that framework, the state can set the income standards from its current Medicaid level up to 200 percent of the federal poverty level. Eligibility can vary by age, residency, geographic area, access to other insurance, and disability status. A family can be covered if the cost of an employer-based family plan is cheaper than covering just the children under CHIP and if the state has obtained a waiver to cover the family. In that case, the state pays the employee's share of a premium subsidized by an employer.

Once again, states had more options than they did with Medicaid but still fewer than they wanted. States gained some narrow flexibility to pass along some of the costs to Medicaid recipients, either through monthly premiums and/or copayments. Cost sharing, or what families are required to pay out of pocket, is restricted to the very low levels allowed by Medicaid states for families under 150 percent of the federal poverty level. Cost sharing for families with incomes over 150 percent of the federal poverty level must be capped at 5 percent of family income.[48] Also, if the state chooses to include recipient cost sharing, it must provide public notice and an opportunity for public comment. There can be no cost sharing for wellness services. The U.S. Department of Health and Human Services (not the states) defines wellness services for the purposes of cost sharing. This is another example of flexibility that only goes so far, and it represents a big win for consumer advocates, who made low out-of-pocket costs a big priority.

Financial safeguards restricting state flexibility were supported by both Democrats and Republicans. States must have an approved plan for their new program and demonstrate appropriate expenditures in order to draw down federal funds. There is a 10 percent cap on administrative expenditures, which includes the cost of direct services and outreach. In other words, CHIP is the payer of last resort. If the person is covered by or eligible for Medicaid, Medicare, or other government programs, those programs must pay first. If the child is covered by a private plan, he or she cannot receive CHIP benefits.

Both Democrats and Republicans added provisions to limit state discretion and protect their own policy interests. In the end, the parties agreed that there should be strong financial reporting requirements to protect against fraud and abuse by the states. Mistrust of the states is a bipartisan issue.

CHIP was driven by the policy interests of federal legislators and a sophisticated legislative strategy. The understanding that states were already developing their own programs proved crucial, even though those programs did not actually cover many children. Liberals used the existence of state plans and the promise of state flexibility to expand health insurance coverage for uninsured children across the country.[49] Legislators also co-opted the state-level practice of paying for children's health programs with tobacco taxes. It was a classic hero-against-villain tale, pitting children and their protectors against an increasingly "evil industry of death." That strategy forced a reluctant Republican leadership to place children's health insurance on the legislative agenda—no members of Congress wanted to be targeted by political ads claiming that they voted for "big tobacco" and against children's health—and eventually secured its passage.

Liberals used federalism and flexibility as a tool to broaden support, while the conservative leadership was torn between an ideological predisposition to grant authority to the states and a desire for national fiscal and policy control. Conservatives vacillated between their desire to limit federal programs and their support for covering "deserving" children. States had a direct influence on program design and financing. Governors pushed their agenda through the Republican leadership, with whom they shared many goals. While governors advocated hard for flexibility, advocacy groups fought for a comprehensive benefits package and national quality standards and assurances. The result was a compromise.

Conservative and liberals were quick to drop any ideological notions of federalism when their interests were at stake. The details of the statute and the floor debates show individual members from both parties adding restrictions to the bill. There was bipartisan support to restrict coverage to uninsured children, prevent shifting from private or other public programs to CHIP, require certain data collection and reporting requirements, reduce the possibility of fraud and abuse, and limit administrative costs. CHIP struck a balance between national accountability and state flexibility through a highly political process marked by strategy, compromise, and power struggles. Inelegant as it was, CHIP displayed intergovernmental structures and policy arrangements that expanded comprehensive benefits coverage to millions of uninsured children. National reform and the ACA mirrored some of CHIP's elements, including Medicaid expansion, benefit design through an actuarial equivalent, the inclusion and prohibition of certain benefits, increased national funding, and state flexibility to design new health insurance exchanges. Unlike CHIP, national reform was not bipartisan and did not engage governors early in its development, a fact that could pose some formidable challenges for implementation.

State activities and the tenets of federalism can be used to forward progressive policy at the national level. Historically, states' rights arguments have been used to thwart national policy, and for decades they were especially effective in stalling civil rights protections for African Americans. CHIP demonstrates how state action and federalism can disarm the arguments about "big government" and "socialized medicine" that helped defeat similar programs in the past. Similarly, Massachusetts and other state health care reform efforts provided cover for the passage of national health care reform.

Such state influence on national policy can be seen beyond the health arena. California state fuel efficiency standards for cars led to national action. States are even becoming active in immigration policy, which is ultimately the responsibility of the federal government. Arizona's efforts in 2012 to crack down on undocumented immigrants and a proposed guest worker program in Utah could each eventually affect national immigration policy, which is all but stalled at the federal level.

The efforts in the 1960s and 1970s to inject progressive health and social welfare policy through Washington directly into the national bloodstream are not politically feasible in the current political climate. Activists seeking such changes need to use an inside-out strategy that works at both the state and the federal level. If reformers could make CHIP a reality in the Gingrich era, there's still hope for the reformers of today.

CHAPTER THREE

CHIP:
FEDERALISM AND
RULEMAKING

Laws passed by Congress do not emerge as finished products. Before they can be fully implemented, they have to go through the underappreciated but crucially important process of administrative rulemaking. This phase defines how a law will work in the real world, thereby creating policy. Rulemaking is nearly as important as the legislative process, but it is often ignored. It's not as sexy as the podium-pounding, headline-grabbing battles that can take place in Congress. It is not easy to understand, and it is often relegated to the domain of wonks, insiders, and lawyers. From personal experience I can attest that there is no better cure for insomnia than spending some quality time with the *Federal Register,* in which the rules are published for comment. But to truly understand how policy is made, you have to open up the black box of the rulemaking process to see how it ticks.

The importance of rulemaking was on full display after the passage of CHIP; Clinton administration officials, interest groups, the states, and Congress all influenced the evolution of the program. The input of the executive branch speaks volumes about current and future policy. A very different CHIP rule would have been created under the conservative George W. Bush administration. Similarly, if President Obama had not been reelected, Mitt Romney would have used executive orders and the rulemaking process to begin "on day one" to weaken and, in effect, overturn many elements of the ACA.[1] Opponents of reform would doubtless have written very different rules governing how health exchanges might work, the design of the essential health insurance benefits package, the Medicaid expansion, and a range of critical decisions needed to make reform work. The pen that writes administrative rules is powerful.

After CHIP passed into law, the Centers for Medicare and Medicaid Services was charged with writing the rules and regulations necessary to expand coverage for uninsured children. The process was anything but straightforward. Congress wanted all that was "good": targeting low-income children with no other source of insurance, preventing fraud and abuse, limiting administrative costs, and preventing parents from dropping other coverage, all while providing certain benefits and prohibiting others. This wish list required strong national standards. Congress and President Clinton were also committed to maximum state flexibility, and CMS had to find a way to reconcile those polar-opposite forces.

In the early days of CHIP, CMS worked in close partnership with the states. But over time, that partnership essentially fell apart under the weight of the federal government. The shift to federal dominance was driven by the requirements of the formal rulemaking process, CMS's sense of mission, and the administration's priorities. In the end, CMS regulations provided national protections at the cost of state autonomy. Lessons for national health care reform include the need to work in partnership with the states to kick-start the program as quickly as possible. The CHIP rulemaking process also demonstrated that state flexibility can be harnessed to reach national health insurance coverage goals but that the process is not likely to be pretty.

INFORMAL RULEMAKING

Proposed CHIP regulations were not written until well after the states began putting the program into action.[2] States could begin receiving CHIP money just two months after the program was signed into law on August 5, 1997. That may seem unusually fast, but it is actually par for the course. Congress generally takes a long time to pass legislation, but when it finally acts, it wants the law implemented immediately. Needless to say, CMS could not possibly complete all of the necessary rules and regulations in such a short time frame. Formal rulemaking requires analysis of implementation options, including cost implications, publication in the *Federal Register*, opportunity for public comment, and a strict process for maintaining public records. That takes time and resources.[3]

In order to meet ambitious deadlines, CMS proposed expedited regulations that would go into effect immediately and allow states to draw down CHIP money. Simultaneously, CMS developed a model template for states to use to submit plans for their new CHIP programs, issued a series of twenty-three letters for state health officials ("Dear State Health Official" letters), published answers to over 100 frequently asked questions, and provided technical assistance to individual states. CMS staff worked tirelessly to get the program up and running, an effort that kept them from working on the formal rules.[4]

Although the initial rules were drawn up quickly, that informal rulemaking process still included a series of bureaucratic checkpoints. All public documents needed to be cleared by a special steering committee, co-chaired by Debbie Chang from CMS and Earl Fox from the Health Resources and Services Administration (HRSA). All the letters, questions and answers, state plans, and state plan amendments had to be approved by CMS, HRSA, and the finance and policy staffs of Secretary of Health and Human Services (HHS) Donna Shalala. Next, documents had to be cleared by the Office of Management and Budget (OMB) and senior White House health policy staff. CMS also held extensive meetings with state and other stakeholders, including child advocacy groups, insurance companies, and provider groups. If states did not like the answers that they received, they could appeal directly to the secretary or to their congressional delegation. It was not exactly a blueprint for a smooth, efficient operation, but it did get the program off the ground.

At that stage, time pressure forced CMS and state officials to cooperate closely in order to resolve problems quickly. Chang characterized the early relationship with the states as collaborative, and her assessment was confirmed by people from the National Governors Association (NGA) and the National Conference of State Legislators (NCSL). As Chang herself noted, states had three avenues for providing direct input into the process: states had direct access to her and her staff to ask questions and express concerns; states had the opportunity to comment on Dear State Health Official letters; and, in particular, CMS negotiated CHIP plans separately with each state. CMS took states' questions and comments and its own responses seriously.

In the early implementation stage, CMS provided significant support to states, including immediate technical assistance.[5] Much of the early work focused on the Medicaid options, the waiver program, and the arrangements of a particular state.[6] Chang noted that because of the close working relationship with the states, "we knew what kind of issues they had, and so we knew what kind of policy questions we had to answer."[7] While states did not get everything that they wanted, they had input into the process, both in negotiating their individual plans and in making comments on proposed national policy.

CMS held periodic briefings with Democratic and Republican congressional staff on Capitol Hill. Soon, the feds took charge. Congress started complaining that CMS was not complying with the CHIP law and eventually requested a detailed accounting of progress at public hearings. Congress, controlled by the Republicans, was concerned that the law was being interpreted too liberally by the Clinton administration. The Republicans were especially concerned that CMS was allowing for family coverage and wanted to make sure that program funds were directed specifically at poor children; they also wanted to prevent people from shifting from Medicaid or private plans to the CHIP program. A senior staff person at NCSL described an unusually aggressive Congress that was "breathing down the neck" of CMS.[8] The House Commerce Committee even published a CHIP implementation guide for the states that summarized the legislation and highlighted the benefits and the flexibility of states to create their own programs.[9] Congress was pushing in two different directions—toward both state flexibility and federal accountability—and CMS was caught in the middle.

Chang left to become Medicaid director for the state of Maryland in June 1998. At that point, a draft of the proposed regulations, based largely on the questions and answers that CMS developed for informal state guidance, had been cleared by CMS and sent to the Office of Management and Budget for review. Chang had been resolute about not renegotiating issues that were resolved in earlier discussions.[10] However, after her departure, the floodgates opened, and the rule was sent back to CMS. A redrafted proposal was issued in November 1999. Relations between CMS and the states deteriorated, a schism that was reflected in harsh comments from the states. The process shifted from partnership to federal control. The rulemaking process became more formal and offered less possibility of direct negotiation with the states. While early attention was given to a flurry of activities to get programs started, CMS became focused more on the policy details of implementation. Since the CMS leadership was no longer operating in crisis mode, it could take a longer, deeper approach to rulemaking, drawing on the Medicaid systems that it knew so well.

FORMAL RULEMAKING

In developing the formal rules, CMS embraced its role as referee, leaving the states to feel like mere players.[11] The states wanted to be treated like sovereign entities, with statutory authority to develop and run the programs,[12] but that is not what they got. A top official from Florida commented: "We believe that CMS initially interpreted and acted upon Congress' and the President's intent correctly. The proposed [formal] regulation takes a major step away from that commitment by stifling innovation and attempting to force the states in to a 'one size fits all' model."[13] Other states weighed in with complaints of their own:

—"Cumbersome and unnecessary" (Georgia).

—"Far exceeds the congressional statute and has no basis in practical wisdom" (Utah).

—"Administrative funds are insufficient to effectively operate a state plan under the proposed regulations" (Wisconsin).

—Enrollment and screening requirements are "taken to the extreme" (Alabama).

—The proposed rule requires "major rethinking" (California).

—"Unduly burdensome," "stringent," and "prescriptive" (Kentucky).

Nearly all the states claimed that the proposal went beyond the authority granted in the statute and imposed unnecessary administrative burdens. In a representative statement, Virginia said that the regulations "restrict the options available to the states, and pressure states into implementing programs that look as much like Medicaid as possible."[14] Several states claimed that the proposal went against President Clinton's executive order on federalism, which mandated that "the national government shall grant to the state the maximum administrative discretion possible."[15]

Meetings of the National Governors Association and the National Conference of State Legislatures gave state representatives fresh chances to express their concerns. A senior health staff person at NGA observed, "Whenever there is a standard that CMS had to develop, they used the default standard of Medicaid, and that can create a large problem for states in terms of how they implement the program."[16] The consensus at the NGA was that the CMS had overstepped its bounds and hampered the ability of states to create their own programs. Attendees at the NCSL bemoaned "punitive" enforcement measures, hefty administrative costs, the inclusion of a consumer bill of rights, "arbitrary" cost sharing, and "biased" crowd-out provisions.[17]

While states pushed for flexibility to create their own programs, advocacy groups pushed for Medicaid-like protections. Groups such as the Children's Defense Fund and Families USA wanted to use CHIP to help streamline the Medicaid program and bring more people into it. They wanted the application process to be simple and straightforward. They wanted safeguards to ensure due process—making it easy to obtain benefits and difficult to take them away. Yet those goals, safeguards, and national protections detracted from state discretion and autonomy. These groups had strong supporters in the White House and in CMS, including Secretary of Health and Human Services Donna Shalala and First Lady Hillary Rodham Clinton.

ANALYSIS OF THE PROPOSED RULE

To really understand how CHIP played out, it is necessary to take a close look at its key elements: eligibility requirements, benefits package, reporting requirements, screening and enrollment, outreach, payment levels, and cost sharing. It quickly becomes clear that it is extremely difficult to layer a new program over and include it within a complex public and private health care system that has evolved over time. National reform will face many of the same challenges. The history of CHIP shows how administrative agencies use the systems that they know, leverage the resources that they have, and reflect the priorities of the administration that they work for in creating policy rules and regulations.

Eligibility

At first, it seemed that states would have wide flexibility in determining eligibility, but that autonomy quickly vanished as the federal government targeted especially needy children. States had plenty of initial reason for optimism. The law allowed them to define what did and what did not count as income; for example, they could choose to use family gross or net income.[18] Further, CMS let the states decide what constituted a family.[19] States could also establish separate standards for different groups of children based on "geographic area served by the plan, age, income, and resources . . . residency, disability status . . . access to other health coverage and duration of eligibility."[20]

However, as the CHIP rule evolved, the states' power to define eligibility dwindled. The new statute directly and indirectly restricted eligibility. Direct restrictions included mandates to cover certain children and not others, to cover low-income before higher-income children, to instate waiting periods, and so forth. The federal government also established residency requirements, rules for treatment of immigrants, the definition of income, civil rights protections, and disability protections under the Americans with Disabilities Act (ADA). Each of those provisions taken separately was reasonable and still provided room for state flexibility, but taken as a whole, they significantly curtailed state autonomy.

Above all, the federal government wanted to target low-income children. The statute required that family incomes must be at or below 200 percent of the poverty line, although some states could raise the bar a little higher.[21] At the lower end, children who were eligible for Medicaid were not allowed in the CHIP program. States were also restricted from covering children with higher incomes without covering those with lower incomes first. In addition, states that chose to run their own programs could not make eligibility for their Medicaid program more restrictive than it was on June 1, 1997; that restriction was to prevent states from shifting people from their Medicaid program to the CHIP program in order to receive the higher federal matching payments.[22] The rule also required parents who dropped children from their health insurance coverage to wait six months before enrolling them in the CHIP program in order to discourage them from dropping their private insurance to join the CHIP program.

States were also restricted by a host of other laws and court rulings. For example, states had to comply with Immigration and Naturalization Service (INS) rules on citizenship following the Personal Responsibility and Work Opportunity Act of 1996, which prohibited new immigrants from receiving benefits for five years.[23] (This prohibition was dropped as part of national health care reform in 2010.) Eligibility criteria also had to comply with civil rights assurances, including compliance with the Civil Rights Act of 1964, the Americans with Disabilities Act of 1990, the Rehabilitation Act of 1973, and the Age Discrimination Act of 1975.[24] Further, eligibility based on residency requirements was limited by the Supreme Court decision in *Shapiro* v. *Thompson,* which prohibited waiting periods on new arrivals to the state. So much for simplifying the eligibility systems.

CMS tried to wedge the program between Medicaid and private insurance, an untidy process to say the least. Still, the process largely works: CHIP children generally come from working families that are not poor enough to be eligible for Medicaid but cannot afford private insurance. Rulemaking for national reform will face similar challenges, on steroids. ACA rules will have to deal with eligibility transitions: people moving between Medicaid, CHIP, subsidized insurance through new health care exchanges, and unsubsidized private or employer-sponsored insurance, depending on changes in their income and family circumstances.

Benefits

In a similar pattern, CHIP regulations initially promised the states considerable flexibility in setting benefits, but state benefit packages became limited by a number of federal requirements, mandates, and safeguards. Similar to the ACA, CHIP must provide a benefits package equivalent to that of a typical "benchmark" plan, perhaps the Federal Employees Health Benefits Program plan, the Blue Cross Blue Shield standard option benefit plan, or the HMO plan in the state that is the most popular in the commercial market (excluding Medicaid enrollment in that HMO).[25] In estimating plan equivalence, state actuaries must meet federal standards and use federal criteria.[26]

The rule stipulates that the plan must include coverage for inpatient and out-patient hospital services, physicians' services, surgical and medical services, laboratory and x-ray services, immunizations, and well-baby and well-child care. Variations in coverage for prescription drugs and mental health, vision, and hearing services were allowed.

Sometimes the statute was clear about its requirements. For example, the Hyde Amendment restricted coverage for abortion unless performed to save the life of the mother or in cases of rape or incest. The rule required abortion services to be paid for entirely by state money from a separate plan—not CHIP.

Such funding restrictions caused problems for certain states with premium assistance programs, which subsidize employer-sponsored insurance for people eligible for Medicaid or CHIP. Massachusetts and New Jersey argued that it did not make sense to take abortion services out if an employer plan already included them.[27] Other specific requirements include having "guarantee[d] access to emergency services without any requirements for prior authorization"[28] and having emergency room services available outside of the plan.[29] All of those provisions set national standards and reduced state flexibility.

Even in areas where the statute was unclear, the power to make policy choices fell mostly to the CMS. For example, CMS requires coverage of well-baby and well-child care. And while states are allowed to define what such care includes, their decisions are subject to CMS approval. CMS further reduced state autonomy by mandating the use of the schedule of the Advisory Committee on Immunization Practice for childhood vaccinations.[30] A number of states objected to such micromanagement. For example, California wanted to continue to use a schedule adopted by the American Academy of Pediatrics and the American Academy of Family Physicians.[31]

States also objected to the fact that CHIP children were not eligible for the 100 percent federally funded "free" vaccines from the Vaccines for Children Program. Here the states wanted CHIP to act more like Medicaid, which does not ask states to pay anything for vaccines. Kentucky stated, "We oppose the arbitrary distinction that denies stand-alone programs access to the Vaccines for Children program."[32] Consumer groups believed that CMS should have defined well-baby and well-child care very broadly. CMS sided with the child advocacy groups and supported universal standards that gave states few options.

In the end, the rule provided some flexibility within a framework of a fairly comprehensive benefit plan. It also included some very specific state requirements. The regulations read, "In approving state child health plans, we intend to ensure that children receive services that are cost effective, comprehensive, and high quality."[33] That prevented states from offering reduced-benefit plans and implied a national standard for a full-service plan. Whenever the CHIP legislation was clear and direct, the rulemaking process followed suit. Where the law was ambiguous, CMS leaned toward Medicaid standards. Likewise, national reform requires federal officials to establish an essential benefits package and then fill in the details of ambiguous legislation. If CHIP is any indication, it's safe to assume that national reform will be a messy affair.

State Plans, Amendments, and Reports

Data collection and reporting requirements in the CHIP rule were substantial and provided considerable information to CMS about state programs, in major contrast to the Health Insurance Portability and Accountability Act (HIPAA). To begin, states were required to collect data on the insurance status of children and document efforts already taken by the state to cover uninsured children. States were also responsible for providing an outline of efforts to coordinate CHIP with their other efforts to expand health care coverage to children.[34] States had to classify children by family income, age, race, and insurance type. Annual reports had to include information on performance measures that were "objective, independent, and verifiable." Each state was required to define strategic objectives, performance goals, and performance measures.[35] States had to make details of program expenditures available and submit them to federal audit, and CMS used the information to ensure that states were meeting core program requirements.

Screening and Enrollment

Screening and enrolling children in CHIP was complicated by the prohibition against letting Medicaid-eligible children into the program, a restriction included to prevent states from shifting kids from Medicaid to CHIP to get bigger payouts from the federal government. To make it easier to see which children were eligible for which program, states were urged to use the same applications for both Medicaid and CHIP.[36] CMS declared that "if a state is using separate applications, DHHS will pay special attention during the review process to the procedures established by the state in order to insure that the 'screen and enroll' requirement is met." In the world of government agencies, the promise of "special attention" is essentially a threat. CMS also required the states to provide prospective CHIP recipients with "full and complete" information about Medicaid, including benefit and cost-sharing differences between the state's Medicaid and CHIP programs.[37]

States believed that this close association to the Medicaid program was antithetical to the original statute. Utah expressed concern that the proposed rule forced states to treat "CHIP applicants as Medicaid applicants."[38] Alabama wrote that the rule had taken the screening and enrollment process for CHIP "to the extreme."[39] Consumer and provider groups, on the other hand, believed that the CHIP law required a full Medicaid screen for every child.[40] Advocates wanted to make sure that if a child was eligible for Medicaid's more comprehensive benefits, he or she received them.[41] In the CHIP law, Congress wanted states to both streamline eligibility for CHIP and exclude children who could be getting Medicaid. But that was like trying to put five gallons of water in a one-gallon drum. In the end, the processes for determining eligibility for both Medicaid and CHIP were simplified, and the result was that both programs ended up covering more children—an ugly process but arguably a good outcome.

Consumer Protections

President Clinton further complicated things for the states by applying his Directive for Consumer Protections to the CHIP program. In other words, he used the rulemaking process to achieve the sort of patient protections that he had failed to achieve through Congress with the Patient Protection Act of 1998.[42] Even supporters of those protections might feel uneasy about such use of executive power, which can cut both ways; it could just as easily be deployed against the best interests of consumers and the general public. Indeed, President George W. Bush used his executive power to significantly reduce eligibility for CHIP.

As part of President Clinton's consumer protection directive, the CHIP rule included the following provisions:

—Information must be given to recipients after enrollment in easily understood language and in a format accessible to the visually impaired and to individuals with limited reading proficiency and language barriers.

—Information must include procedures for obtaining services, authorization requirements, availability of after-hours and emergency care, cost-sharing requirements, and complaint, grievance, and fair hearing procedures.

—There must be choice of health plan and provider.

—Access to specialists must be ensured.

—Access to emergency room services must be guaranteed.

—Patients must have the opportunity to participate in treatment decisions.

—States must establish procedures for providing conflict-of-interest information on physicians' financial arrangements that could affect treatment decisions.

—Patient confidentiality must be protected, and beneficiaries must have the right to review all documentation.[43]

Those federal requirements forced states to change their administrative and operating procedures. Although most of the states had consumer protection laws, some better than those proposed, the states still objected that the CMS was exceeding its statutory authority.[44]

Payment Levels

The proposed regulations made it clear that states determined the payment levels for providers. However, in the section on fraud and abuse, CMS required the states to "set rates in a manner that most efficiently utilizes limited CHIP funds."[45] More specifically, the CMS required that fee-for-service rates should be based on public and private payment rates for comparable services, unless higher rates were necessary to attract providers in underserved areas. CMS at least reserved the right to compare payment rates against identified criteria. While the section on payments provided flexibility, other sections of the law took it away.

Cost Sharing

In a recurring pattern, states gained some leeway in setting cost sharing, but they also found their hands tied in significant ways. First, cost sharing—which covers enrollment fees, premiums, deductibles, copayments, and coinsurance—could not be done in a way that favored children from higher-income families. Second, total beneficiary costs were capped at 5 percent of income for families with an income of more than 150 percent of the federal poverty level and at 2.5 percent of income for families with income under that line.[46] Third, cost sharing was prohibited for well-baby and well-child care, as defined by CMS. Fourth, by statute, no cost sharing was allowed for American Indians and Alaska Natives.

There were a number of additional federal safeguards for people with incomes of less than 150 percent of the poverty line. Premiums were restricted to those allowed under Medicaid, which are nominal. The plan could not include more than one type of cost sharing, which meant that a person paying a deductible could not also be charged a copayment. Only one copayment could be charged for multiple procedures during a single visit. The maximum copayment was set at $5.00, up from $3.00 for Medicaid. The maximum deductible was $3.00, up from $2.00 for Medicaid. Further, a maximum of only $10 could be charged for non-emergency use of an emergency room.

States have more flexibility to determine cost-sharing rules for families with incomes of more than 150 percent of the federal poverty level; they are far less trusted with setting cost sharing for families under that line. States strongly objected to federal cost-sharing requirements. Most believed the 2.5

percent cap was arbitrary and noted that it was not mentioned in the statute. CMS came up with this arrangement to implement the statute's requirement that lower-income recipients not pay costs that were greater relative to those of higher-income recipients. States were also concerned about the administrative cost of tracking out-of-pocket expenses, especially since reports indicated that only a small percentage of participants would ever exceed the cap and have to pay anything out of pocket.

States further objected that CMS defined dental services, routine physician's visits, and lab tests as well as well-baby and well-child care for the purpose of cost sharing. States believed that this cost structure would discourage their CHIP programs from offering these benefits. States were also nearly unanimous in their objection to waiving the cost-sharing requirement for American Indians and Alaska Natives. Noting the difficulty of segmenting populations and targeting benefits, they objected to the administrative complexity of the requirement. States pointed out that no other provisions in the statue were modified on the basis of race or ethnicity. Several states made the suggestion that since the federal government was obligated to meet the health needs of this group, it should pay 100 percent of the cost.

Cost sharing was a major issue for child advocates, the Clinton administration, and those within CMS, who viewed it as a possible barrier to coverage and services. They agreed that very few people would reach the caps but pointed out that the people that did were more likely to have significant disabilities and require more services.[47] States that created their own program or used existing commercial products were constrained by the cost-sharing requirements. In this trade-off, national consumer protection was again favored over state autonomy.

Congress gave CMS and the states an impossible timetable for getting CHIP up and running, resulting in a lot of scrambling to bring the program on line. The initial phase was characterized by relatively open communication and partnership between the agency and the states. However, the CHIP rulemaking process became increasingly formal and restrictive as political attention waned and the initial pressure to get the program started subsided, and what was initially seen as a partnership between states and the CMS was eventually overshadowed by national control of the process. The proposed CHIP rule demonstrated tension between universal goals and requirements and a commitment to state flexibility and program diversity. For example, although states were given discretion to set eligibility requirements, those requirements had to comply with various federal rules: they needed to make sure that they did not cover children eligible for Medicaid or any other source of care, and they needed to comply with other federal laws, court cases, and executive orders.

The politics and interests of the White House, congressional oversight, interest group pressure, and the concerns of the CMS officials writing the regulations directly influenced the design and shape of the CHIP law after passage. Congress was far more active in the period immediately after the law was passed but then moved on to other priorities. The rulemaking process was an ongoing political struggle to clarify ambiguity in the statute, and it even added provisions, like the patient's bill of rights, that were not in the statute. Again, a very different program could have emerged if the rule were written by a different administration with different priorities.

In this way, presidential elections directly influence how programs are ultimately shaped and structured. If CHIP rules had been written during the George W. Bush administration, states would have been given more power—for example, to limit benefit plans. Consumer protection would have been left up to the states. States would have had more options to reduce program costs by charging beneficiaries higher premiums.

With a deeper understanding of the importance of the rulemaking process, it should be clear how important the reelection of President Obama was to sustaining the ACA. In 2012, the House voted to repeal the law and continues to threaten to hold up funding for rulemaking and implementation. Presidential contender Romney campaigned against the ACA. Meanwhile, the Obama administration worked as quickly as possible to write regulations and put as many stakes in the ground as possible to protect its legislative accomplishment. However, implementation of the ACA is to occur over a long period, with critical elements not coming on line until 2014 and some stretching beyond that. The CHIP experience suggests that the administration should continue to expedite the regulation process and work collaboratively with the states to get the program up and running as quickly as possible. Rules and regulations define a program and make it real. The alternatives are to allow existing ambiguities to remain, which would weaken the program, or to let it be defined by the next administration, the states, or the courts. Through their comments and political access to the administration, providers, consumers, and business and other interests also can have a real and direct impact on the rules.

The CHIP rulemaking process demonstrated that it is possible to allow state flexibility within federally defined corridors. It is possible for states to adapt health insurance reforms to local markets and private sector offerings and still target the uninsured with a comprehensive benefits package. The degree of federal control or flexibility depends on political pressure, previously institutionalized programs, congressional interests, and the priorities of the administration.

CHAPTER FOUR

CHIP:
FEDERALISM AND
IMPLEMENTATION

Implementation is where the rubber hits the road, where abstract policies and rules have real impacts on people, where intergovernmental relations are solidified in practice. As a process, implementation turns out to be every bit as political as rulemaking. Analysis of CHIP implementation reveals that in a collaborative effort to make the program work, broader national safeguards remained even as states regained some autonomy. The federal government negotiated directly with different states, which led to variations throughout the country. Despite some inconsistencies, CHIP accomplished its main goals: to provide public health insurance to eligible children and to reduce the disparities in public coverage, which was an important concern. How that happened provides insight into the health policy process and offers lessons for the implementation of national reform.

After a slow start, implementation of CHIP was a success. In March 1997, only four states provided coverage for all children whose household incomes were less than 200 percent of the federal poverty level (FPL); by January 2000, thirty states provided coverage for all children under that level and five states for children up to or over 300 percent of the FPL.[1] Prior to CHIP, only eleven states offered coverage to children living in households whose income was above 185 percent of the FPL; by 2007, forty-two states offered coverage to children up to or over 200 percent of the FPL.[2] Those numbers add up to an important message: CHIP worked.

As CHIP programs came on line, the enrollment procedures, eligibility rules, benefits, and cost-sharing provisions that emerged were remarkably consistent—much more so than could have been expected if the states had broad flexibility to set their own terms. CHIP also had an unanticipated effect on the Medicaid program: it streamlined the eligibility process and increased enrollment. The balance between flexibility and greater national uniformity was achieved by a combination of CMS regulations (the stick) and enhanced federal funding (the carrot). Strictly applying universal standards to different baseline state systems and programs does not work. Flexibility is the grease that makes the system run.

While CMS and the states ultimately found a balance between federal standards and state flexibility, the process was not easy. The two sides approached the task from different perspectives—CMS was concerned with national policy while the states were preoccupied with local politics, markets, and operational details—and that made communication difficult and frustrating. Still, the two sides managed to create a relationship through bargaining and negotiation, although CMS did dictate some standards. CMS dug in on particular issues, like cost sharing and giving priority to covering low-income children, when faced with pressure from Congress, the administration, or interest groups. Negotiations took center stage when solutions were unclear and resolution was in the interest of both parties.

These findings foreshadow the opportunities and challenges for national reform; they also hint at potential unanticipated consequences. Simply boosting federal funding for Medicaid expansions and for health care exchanges will not be enough. Political opposition at the state level can slow, stall, or completely prevent reform, but opposition can be quieted by early success and a greater awareness among federal officials of the challenges that states face. States will need flexibility to make national reform work; the federal government cannot expect Texas to follow the same rules as Rhode Island. Unanticipated consequences may include larger enrollment in the traditional Medicaid program and higher-than-predicted state costs. Implementation is always difficult, and creating new administrative systems only increases the challenge. The longer time horizon for implementing national reform prolongs the pain, much as slowly pulling a Band-Aid off a cut does. Implementation is a political as well as technical undertaking, and success will be determined by elections, politicians, and the availability and use of resources.

STATE PROGRAMS

In the first year of CHIP, CMS quickly approved plans submitted by the states and territories. The majority of states (twenty-six) simply expanded their Medicaid program, but over time more states created separate programs.[3] Enrollment in the first year was slow, and the fifty states ended up covering fewer than 830,000 children, well below expectations.[4] Even toward the end of the second year (October 1, 1999), three states (Hawaii, Washington, and

Wyoming) had yet to enroll a single child.[5] The Congressional Budget Office estimated that the states spent only one-quarter of their allotment in year two (FY 1999). Supporters in the White House, Congress, and advocacy organizations were concerned that the program was not meeting enrollment targets.[6]

Unreasonable expectations helped set the stage for the slow start. A senior official at the National Conference of State Legislatures (NCSL) explained it well: "Programs are often oversold to build consensus for them in Congress, and then the states have to appropriate money, redesign policies, reeducate eligibility workers, and redo forms." She noted that "it took a good 10 years for Medicare to mature as a program."[7] New programs and systems have to be designed and adjusted before the process of winning approval of state legislatures can even begin, and each step takes time. Similar systems and infrastructure will need to be created as national health care reform comes on line.

A Slow Start

A study of early implementation in six states with especially solid systems for insuring children showed that even those states had trouble spending their first year's allotment.[8] A number of states claimed that even if they had fully operational programs and 100 percent participation, it would not be possible to spend all of the CHIP money. An Urban Institute report concluded that only 30 percent of all uninsured children were actually eligible for the CHIP program.[9] In other words, 3.2 million children were eligible for a program funded to cover 6 million. The report rightly predicted that the states would have a hard time spending all their money.[10]

As it turned out, more uninsured children were actually eligible for Medicaid than were eligible for CHIP. So why weren't they already enrolled in Medicaid? The reasons were the same as those that always keep potential beneficiaries from their benefits: confusion over eligibility (particularly in light of welfare reform changes that were going on at that time), complex eligibility rules and documentation requirements, the stigma associated with a welfare program, and language and cultural barriers.[11] In addition, many low-income parents need to set priorities for meeting basic needs, and buying health insurance for apparently healthy children may not take priority; only when a child becomes ill or is injured does the need for health insurance become clear.

In total, 45 percent of the $4.2 billion dollars allocated for FY 1998 went unspent.[12] Forty states did not spend their first-year allotment. Notably, New York was one of the few states able to spend all of its CHIP money in the first year;[13] in fact, this single state accounted for 25 percent of program expenditures in the first few years. However, New York was playing fast and loose with the rules: more than half of the children covered in New York's program were actually eligible for Medicaid. The state was subsequently reprimanded and had to repay a portion of its CHIP money.

A CMS official summed up the mood as states struggled to make the most of CHIP: "Many of the states were surprised at how complicated and time consuming the undertaking was."[14] The *New York Times* interviewed twenty state officials and asked them why they did not spend their allotment. They gave the following reasons:

—slow startup
—reluctance to put up the state's share of the funds
—insufficient number of eligible children to spend all the money allocated
—complex application and enrollment procedures
—rigid, inflexible federal administration.[15]

California and Texas accounted for more than half of the unspent money, despite great needs in each state.[16] The Texas legislature did not meet until January 1999, and the state was late in developing a substantial proposal. California got off to a slow start, too, partly because of foot-dragging under a conservative administration. California also had a complex, twenty-eight-page Medicaid application, which made it that much more difficult to determine which children were eligible for which program.[17] Minnesota spent less than $500,000 of its $28.4 million, but for a different reason. Before CHIP, Minnesota had already covered children with household incomes of up to 275 percent of the FPL through its Medicaid program.[18]

State politics affected CHIP despite strong bipartisan support for the program. National health reform will be similarly buffeted by state-level politics and the whims of legislatures. While national reform will be rolled out over a longer time horizon, initial opposition was more intense than it ever was with CHIP. As a result, many states are unlikely to do anything until they are forced to act.

MEDICAID EXPANSION

While the states had opposed Medicaid expansion in Congress, at first many states opted to expand Medicaid rather than create a new CHIP program. An important consideration was that CHIP gave states an opportunity to level eligibility rules across age and income categories. Previously, many states had covered younger children at higher levels of income than older children. Similarly, national reform increases Medicaid eligibility for adults having incomes of up to 133 percent of the federal poverty level regardless of whether they are disabled or meet any other eligibility standard, and it does so primarily with federal money. That has the possibility of creating a solid safety net at the bottom of the income scale and leveling income eligibility across the country. While this is far from the universal safety net provided by other industrialized nations, it would be a major step for the United States. The CHIP experience suggests that existing state infrastructure will make this provision relatively easy to implement, as long as states receive adequate federal funding.

With CHIP, states that had opposed expanding Medicaid soon found out that in the short run, it was simpler than creating a new program.[19] Medicaid agencies also are more powerful than most state agencies, so they tend to win turf battles. Christie Ferguson, former director of human services for Rhode Island, said that even in a good economy, there is very little interest in increasing the size of state bureaucracies.[20] Legislators are quite willing to give existing bureaucracies more responsibilities, but they resist adding new permanent employees. States prefer, as does CMS, to build on existing systems and infrastructure, working with what they have and what they know. National reform will provide initial startup funding for states to explore options for creating health exchanges. That will certainly help, but building new programs, especially in times of economic hardship, will take time and resources. Success will depend largely on the level of support and the effort of state officials.

BUILDING ON SUCCESS

Over time, more and more states created their own CHIP programs, and after two years momentum began to build. At that point, all states had approved programs and 2 million new children were covered; approximately 1.3 million were enrolled in CHIP and 700,000 were enrolled in Medicaid expansions.[21] The increased enrollment was made possible through concerted outreach efforts that were funded by the federal government and supported by state governors. CHIP increasingly became viewed as a success. By September 1999, forty-five states had expanded income eligibility for infants, forty-nine had expanded coverage for children between the ages of one and six years, and all fifty states had expanded coverage for children between the ages of six and fifteen.[22] Governors bragged about the number of children covered, and members of Congress from both parties cited their support for CHIP when they ran for office in 2000.[23]

DIVERSITY OF STATE PROGRAMS

As expected, states that took the opportunity to build their own programs came up with systems that were different from each other and from Medicaid. But they had a common motivation: they were primarily interested in having insurance programs that resembled those in the private sector. States with stand-alone programs also believed that they could reduce the welfare stigma associated with the Medicaid program, reduce costs, and help build more positive relationships with providers.[24] Maryland, for example, calculated that it would be cheaper and more feasible to create a new program than to expand Medicaid. Savings were attributed to streamlined administration and a less-generous benefits package.[25] The differences and similarities of these stand-alone programs in terms of enrollment, eligibility, benefits, and cost sharing illustrate the importance of giving states the flexibility to adapt to unique environments.

ENROLLMENT AND ELIGIBILITY

The slow pace of early enrollment focused the state and national efforts to improve outreach and streamline eligibility procedures. CHIP proponents were concerned that limited enrollment would diminish long-term support for the program, and that prospect led CMS to encourage the states to move toward adopting a uniform and simpler eligibility system for both the Medicaid and CHIP programs. All but one state in the Government Accountability Office (GAO) fifteen-state sample streamlined the eligibility process by easing eligibility requirements, providing for up to twelve months of continuous eligibility, and/or creating a shorter or joint application form for CHIP and Medicaid.[26] Still, considerable diversity in eligibility remained among states, in large part because state-based Medicaid programs differed so much. The GAO reported that "[data] comparisons across states will be difficult because of differences in eligibility standards [and in] the definition and categorization of income."[27]

An unexpected result of CHIP was that the combined, streamlined applications boosted enrollment in Medicaid. Nationwide, an average of one child was found eligible for Medicaid for every child found eligible for CHIP.[28] Massachusetts found two children eligible for Medicaid for every one found eligible for CHIP.[29] Similarly, national reform—especially when coupled with an individual insurance mandate—should lead to a substantial increase in Medicaid enrollment, which could place a considerable burden on state budgets.

States used flexibility to define income and expand eligibility beyond the official CHIP ceiling. For example, Connecticut disregarded certain types of income to move effective eligibility from 185 percent to 300 percent of FPL, and New York took a similar approach, effectively moving the bar to 222 percent of FPL. CMS supported such adjustments.[30] Some states took advantage of flexibility to keep children in the program longer despite changes in family income. By the end of January 2000, eighteen states had continuous CHIP coverage for twelve months regardless of income fluctuations, while fourteen states adopted continuous coverage for Medicaid recipients.[31] CMS encouraged state flexibility in determining eligibility to expand the number of children covered and to lengthen the duration of coverage.

OUTREACH

The Clinton administration helped orchestrate and fund a major outreach initiative. In February 1998, President Clinton created the Interagency Children's Health Outreach Taskforce, which included eight federal agencies. Congress included a line item in its budget that increased the ability of states to use welfare reform money to do outreach for health-related programs. In 1999, Congress and the administration allowed states to use $500 million from welfare reform to increase outreach efforts for the CHIP program.[32] The National Governors Association (NGA) joined with CMS to create a national toll-free hotline that directed people to programs in their state. States developed a number of innovative approaches to outreach, and CMS helped publicize the best practices. The emphasis on outreach and corresponding state action helped turn around the disappointing first-year enrollment. Similar innovations in outreach were critical to Massachusetts reform efforts, and they will be essential for national reform to make major inroads on covering the uninsured. The question is whether there will be political support within the states and enough intergovernmental support to conduct the outreach necessary.

BENEFITS

In practice, states implemented comprehensive benefits packages that were more generous than those in the private insurance sector and less generous than Medicaid.[33] In 2000, the Children's Defense Fund reported that forty-three states provided "comprehensive, child-appropriate benefit packages with the same types of benefits covered by Medicaid." Arizona, Delaware,

Montana, and Utah used their state employee benefits package as the standard for CHIP benefits, and Colorado used the standard option in its small group insurance program.[34] An exemption included in the CHIP law allowed Pennsylvania and Florida to keep their pre-CHIP benefits, which were less comprehensive than those of other states. New York had the same exemption but added a number of benefits, including coverage of dental, speech, hearing, and vision (including eyeglasses) services; durable medical equipment; inpatient mental health services; and alcohol and substance abuse treatment.[35]

The GAO report on new state programs concluded that the state benefit levels generally were similar to Medicaid levels, with limits placed on certain services, similar to the limits placed on adults in Medicaid.[36] Connecticut, Florida, and Massachusetts had a benefits package for CHIP recipients similar to those of private plans, but they added a screening and diagnostic benefit that identifies children with behavioral or medical conditions that may require additional benefits.[37] Florida approved an amendment that allows these special CHIP-eligible children to receive Medicaid benefits, and Massachusetts enrolled such children directly in the Medicaid program.[38] States offered most optional services but placed more limits on them than Medicaid did, including restrictions on mental health coverage and vision, dental, and hearing services.[39] Driven by the statute and rule to provide comprehensive benefits, many states went beyond the minimum to offer a number of optional benefits.

Prior to CHIP, state-only programs tended to choose limited benefits packages. With significant federal funding, states opted to provide comprehensive benefits. Most provided optional services with restrictions similar to those of private insurance plans. Some states made additional accommodations for children with special needs. Implementation showed some diversity and innovation but also a high degree of uniformity. Some of that can be attributed to CHIP rules and the desire of states, given the added incentive of federal money, to provide extensive benefits to children. National reform will require health plans to meet minimum essential coverage standards. The gap between those benefits and what the states already offer will largely determine the ease—or difficulty—of implementation.

COST SHARING

The cost-sharing burden on families enrolled in CHIP turned out to be minimal and actually less than allowed by statute.[40] States used cost sharing to reduce the use of unnecessary care, to invoke "personal responsibility," and to avoid displacement of private insurance.[41] All states and private insurers were using the "shoebox approach" (so called because it requires beneficiaries to track their own expenditures and keep all the receipts, as if in a shoebox).[42] Many of the states with stand-alone programs claimed that "the administrative burden of monitoring cost sharing [was] out of proportion to the small amounts of cost sharing actually collected."[43] Only a small portion of children within the state programs had to pay costs that exceeded 5 percent of family income. Advocacy groups point out that while the number over the cap may be small, the children involved often are the most vulnerable, with disabilities or extensive medical costs or both.

Advocacy groups were insistent that cost sharing and premiums be tracked directly by the state (not beneficiaries) and monitored closely to ensure accuracy. Some states addressed this issue by identifying those who used a high level of services and placing them in the Medicaid program (Connecticut, Florida, and Massachusetts). States also used cost sharing to make their programs operate more like private plans. And, like private plan administrators, they found it difficult to track thousands of small transactions. In general, states kept cost sharing to a minimum in part because of tracking difficulties. A survey of a sample of states concluded that "cost-sharing arrangements under CHIP are not a feature that sets new and separate programs significantly apart from Medicaid expansions."[44]

The federal government largely succeeded in promoting flexibility, within constraints that ensured comprehensive coverage with limited out-of-pocket costs. It took oversight, strict reporting requirements, bargaining, and negotiations—yet another lesson for national reform.

CMS-State Relations

My interviews with senior CMS and state officials—primarily in Massachusetts, Rhode Island, and Maryland—shed important light on the relations between the states and the CMS; I also drew on my four years of work at the CMS New England regional office. Understanding CMS-state relations is important because they directly influenced CHIP's development and implementation. CMS's culture, policy perspective, and emphasis on accountability pushed it toward regulating diverse state programs through universal standards. States were concerned about operational systems and how programs would actually work; concerns included issues such as how eligible children would be identified, targeted, and enrolled to obtain health insurance. CMS tended to change policy direction in midstream when officials in Washington shifted priorities, causing significant problems for the states;

they needed lead time to develop operational systems, which are difficult and costly to change. Relationships between CMS and the states during implementation were largely collaborative, but at times CMS set and enforced specific directives without consulting the states.

CMS regional offices monitor state programs and provide technical assistance to explain what the regulations mean, how they apply, and how the state can comply with them. Regional staffs have both specific state and policy expertise and serve as the eyes and ears of the central office in Baltimore, Maryland. Senior state Medicaid officials interviewed in Maryland, Massachusetts, and Rhode Island characterized their experience with the regional office staff as largely collaborative.[45] For example, the CMS regional office provided Rhode Island with technical assistance and lent the state the services of a number of people with backgrounds in Medicaid managed care.

That said, the central office made most of the policy decisions and all of the important ones. The central office negotiated state plans and amendments; when states needed something important, they went directly to the central office. When activities such as monitoring and accounting became routine, they became the responsibility of the regional office. Regional office staff met regularly with state officials and reported back to the central office. When an issue was deemed important, such as a major waiver to Medicaid rules or an egregious case of noncompliance, the central office sent a team for a site visit. Regional offices tended to have a better understanding of the local environment and were often caught between CMS's and the states' differing views of reality. Bruce Bullen, a former Medicaid director, noted that the "central office is trained to set national standards. The regional office is often stuck having to enforce things that it thinks are not right or are inappropriate [given a particular situation in a state], or it is forced to fight back against the central office on behalf of the states."[46]

DIFFERENT PERSPECTIVES

CMS and the states have vastly different agendas and worldviews. CMS's experience is national; it is policy oriented and regulatory. CMS responds to pressure from Congress, the president, senior administrative officials, and national interest groups. Meanwhile, state program directors are concerned with the details of program implementation, which is subject to local political and market pressures. Medicaid and CHIP directors are forced to pay more attention to the logistics of data information systems, staff levels, worker training, the development and disbursement of materials, and negotiations with health plans. Maryland's Medicaid director, who had been a senior CMS official, said that CMS did not have sufficient understanding of the essential link between policy and the systems necessary for implementation. She noted that an agency can have the best policy in the world but that if the systems (management information systems and others) available cannot handle it, it has limited value.[47]

The primary culture in CMS is based on the Medicare program, which is largely centrally directed and administered; the majority of CMS employees work on the Medicare program. States, NGA, and NCSL representatives expressed concern about CMS's tendency to enforce universal standards across diverse state programs.[48] A senior state Medicaid official said, "One cannot turn it [Medicaid and CHIP] into something equivalent to the Medicare program, which is what CMS tries to do too often by issuing regulations to standardize across all 50 states some set of activities."[49] He added that most states would agree that "CMS, particularly central [office], tries to micromanage marketplaces in the states too much."[50] Reasons given include bureaucratic culture, central office domination of policy, staff shortages, and pressure from senior administrative officials, Congress, or interest groups.

All three senior state health officials interviewed agreed that sometimes directives, guidance, or regulations from CMS did not make sense in a given state's particular situation. One said, "It's not because CMS is not trying to do its job. It's because in attempting to apply a policy across all 50 states with 50 programs that are operating in different ways, there is no way that they can issue guidelines that work."[51] Implementation of health exchanges under national health care reform will face a similar challenge in trying to implement a standardized policy over fifty different health care systems; state flexibility at the implementation phase will be required to make it work. Containing and targeting flexibility is required to move toward equalizing the availability of affordable comprehensive health care insurance among states and across the country.

Several senior state officials said that CMS did not have a good understanding of state day-to-day program operations or a sufficient appreciation of the link between policy and system operations. For example, policy changes often require adjustments to the Medicaid Management Information System (MMIS) that can take between six and twelve months to implement.[52] Changing data elements to make reporting more consistent nationwide may not help states run their programs any better, but it can entail significant costs. There is often a difference between what CMS wants and the information necessary to run a program. States complained that Medicaid and CHIP data regularly reported to CMS go into a "black hole" and that they never receive feedback or believe that the information is used in a constructive manner.[53] The constant revision of policies was a real problem for states.[54] CMS dealt with issues as they arose without an appreciation of the cumulative effect on states. States need long lead times to design their infrastructure, information systems, forms, worker training procedures, and contracts with providers. When CMS changes policy, even if the state agrees with the substance, it often entails significant administrative costs with potentially minimal benefits to the state.

State flexibility, however, arose from both lax enforcement and the states' superior knowledge of program details. In other words, states took control when CMS wasn't looking. In speaking with state officials, I realized that the states took their directives from CMS seriously and regarded its authority as legitimate. However, some rules were not enforced, and CMS had clearly shown that it would not shut down a program because it had not followed certain procedures. For example, in the Medicaid program, most states flouted the rule that required federally qualified health centers to be staffed with outstation workers who could process Medicaid applications. A representative from NSCL said that states tried to avoid any battles with CMS that could turn into protracted "paper wars" or messy lawsuits.[55] Generally states tried to meet CMS requirements, directly or through negotiation. But if CMS did not ask for detailed information, the states did not feel compelled to offer it.[56] Where CMS rules are general and their focus is limited, states gain flexibility—the grease to make the programs work.

COMMUNICATION STYLES

At the beginning of the CHIP approval process, communication between the states and CMS focused on bargaining and negotiating. Massachusetts and Rhode Island both spent an exceptional number of hours with CMS negotiating their particular situations. In both cases, a key issue was how the CHIP program would work with the states' Medicaid program and previously federally granted state health care reform waivers and demonstration programs. Massachusetts believed that its recently approved waiver accomplished essentially the same goals as CHIP, meaning that the state should receive its CHIP reimbursement immediately.[57] CMS was initially resistant, and it took hard negotiating to allow the state to incorporate CHIP into the waiver allowing employer subsidies.[58]

Negotiations were not always resolved in the states' favor. In early negotiations over CHIP, Rhode Island failed in its attempt to extend coverage to the parents and other family members of eligible children. Wisconsin experienced similar frustrations. A spokesperson for the Wisconsin Department of Health and Family Services lamented that "at first, the federal officials said they [Wisconsin] could do it that way, but later reneged." He added that "they played games with us for about 18 months."[59] Eventually, both Rhode Island and Wisconsin (along with New Jersey) were among the first states to receive Section 1115 waivers to use CHIP money to cover low-income families.

CMS is quite willing to play the role of enforcer when the need arises. Issues involving accounting and reimbursement—definite priorities for Congress and the White House—are especially likely to make CMS more authoritative and rigid. Christie Ferguson, the former director of human services for Rhode Island, said that federal-state relations were usually based on negotiations, but at times CMS would say, "Here is the rule, and we are going to enforce it." She added, "This happens more at the accounting level, way down low in the bureaucracy."[60]

In hindsight, it is not at all surprising that CHIP got off to a slow start. More resources and effort were needed to educate people about the program. The mid-course correction helped increase participation rates and turned the image of the program around. Diversity exists among state programs (an indication of state autonomy), but it is bound by certain constraints (an indication of federal control). Benefits packages varied, but all were fairly comprehensive. Pre-CHIP state-only programs had a much more diverse range of benefits. CHIP helped level the playing field without trampling state autonomy.

CMS provided flexibility and technical assistance when it was in line with agency, administration, or congressional goals. The differences in policy perspectives among the states tended to frustrate communication, but in the end interactions worked to meet program goals and expand comprehensive health insurance to children in families of low and moderate incomes.

There are many lessons here for the implementation of national reform. CHIP demonstrates that federal money and regulations—together with latitude for state innovation—can make major inroads on covering the uninsured and narrowing coverage gaps between states. ACA's Medicaid expansions will be easiest to achieve because states already have systems in place and the expansions will be financed largely with federal dollars. Creating new health exchanges with tax subsidies will be far more challenging.

CHIP demonstrates that it is possible for the federal government to set coverage and benefit standards as long as states have the flexibility to make adjustments to fit their existing health insurance environment. Uniformity between exchanges can be enhanced by strong reporting requirements and clear federal guidelines and support.

The importance of political support from the state cannot be underestimated. Texas and California were especially slow to start CHIP programs because of their less-than-enthusiastic conservative governors. National reform was passed along partisan lines and poses a far greater political challenge. The House of Representatives voted to repeal the law in 2012, and twenty-seven state attorneys general challenged its constitutionality. Opposing states will continue to resist, as will conservatives in Congress. The chances of success are enhanced by implementing reform as quickly as possible, infusing as much federal money into the system as feasible, and touting early successes. That explains why the Obama administration rapidly dispersed health care exchange and health information technology grants to states in the wake of passage. It also is important for the federal government to work closely with state officials at the staff level and show a clear knowledge of the implementation challenges that they face. Enhancing state flexibility to expedite implementation may mean sacrificing national uniformity, but it will help set a foundation and infrastructure that will root national reform and create a base for further refinement. Conversely, opponents of reform would be wise to slow implementation, reduce resources going to the states, and give states so much discretion that national reform will be unrecognizable. This strategy will rob reform of its roots, and any of its fruits will die on the vine.

CHAPTER FIVE

HIPAA:
FEDERALISM
IN CONGRESS

When I tell my graduate students, "Today we will be talking about something truly fascinating [dramatic pause]: health insurance regulation," the line never fails to elicit groans. The truth is that health insurance can be intriguing—except for the parts that are bone dry. But grasping the complexity of the issue is essential to understanding how the U.S. health care system works and how it might be shaped by national reform.

The Health Insurance Portability and Accountability Act (HIPAA) of 1996—an act that passed in the wake of failed national reform at a time when conservatives controlled Congress—is an important example of health policy in action. HIPAA took aim at some of the most egregious health insurance practices. For example, health insurance companies were allowed to exclude specific body parts from coverage. If Uncle John had a heart murmur and moved from one job to the next, his new insurance company could exempt his heart from coverage; the policy would be literally heartless. That practice led to "job lock"—people staying in jobs that they disliked because changing jobs might mean losing health insurance. Further, insurance companies could drop just individual policies or small group policies to save money. If an employee at a hardware store got AIDS, cancer, or some other devastating, expensive illness, the insurance company could drop coverage for the hardware store at annual renewal. Some people know HIPAA best as the law that establishes privacy standards and protects personal health information, but it sought to accomplish many things. The focus here will be on its efforts to eliminate preexisting condition exclusions and make health insurance more available and affordable. From the beginning, portability was a key issue. In HIPAA, portability does not, as the name suggests, mean keeping the same health plan when one changes jobs; it means that one cannot be

57

denied complete coverage when changing insurance. Studying HIPAA portability provisions and particularly intergovernmental failures to accomplish portability goals offers valuable lessons for the implementation of insurance regulations under the Affordable Care Act.

HIPAA provided minimum national health insurance standards in an area traditionally regulated by the states. While governors influenced CHIP through their political connections with congressional leaders, state insurance commissioners influenced HIPAA through their expertise. For both CHIP and HIPAA, existing state activities were essential precursors to federal action. But unlike with CHIP, the legislative debate over HIPAA had less direct focus on federalism and the arguments that the parties offered ran counter to their conventional stance on states' rights. In this so-called time of "devolution," conservatives supported national regulations that preempted states' rights in order to support business; they were opposed to protecting states' rights when doing so allowed for stronger, more diverse state regulations. Meanwhile, liberals wanted states to have the ability to implement consumer protections that were stronger than the federal government's minimum standards. Positions on federalism were more closely linked to policy interests than to the ideological notions of the "proper" division of power between the states and the federal government.

STATE ACTION

States traditionally have had the power to regulate the small group and individual health insurance markets. Prior to HIPAA, the majority of states had insurance regulations equal to and in most cases stronger than those that HIPAA ultimately included. But states had a problem: they could not regulate the insurance offered by most large employers. Approximately 40 percent of Americans with private insurance are in health insurance plans exempt from state regulation because of a complex labor and pension law called the Employee Retirement Income Security Act of 1974 (ERISA).[1] Those plans are regulated by the federal government, which has traditionally had a far more hands-off approach to regulation than the states. The logic behind the law was that because larger companies have employees in multiple states, it would be burdensome for them to comply with multiple sets of state regulations.

ERISA significantly limited the reach of state insurance regulators. For example, in the 1990s, a number of states passed regulations to prevent hospitals from discharging new mothers within forty-eight hours of birth—so-called "drive-by deliveries." However, such regulations did not apply to larger companies. The same was true for state efforts to limit preexisting condition exclusions and to protect people from "job lock."

Not surprisingly, states were supportive of HIPAA regulations. A key congressional staff member heard directly from the states that "we can only do so much because of ERISA so you all [the federal government] need to do something."[2] Legislators pointed to existing state regulations and programs to gain support for HIPAA. The fact that federal law was often weaker than laws that were already in place in most states helped pave the way for Republican support.[3] While HIPAA expanded insurance regulations, it did not abandon the dual system of state and federal control created by ERISA. ERISA provides businesses protection from state regulations and allows them to more easily offer the same insurance coverage across different states. Labor benefits from ERISA because it protects the health insurance benefits that they have negotiated for over time.[4]

CONGRESS

The Senate and House took different approaches to HIPAA. The bipartisan Senate bill, designed from the beginning to be noncontroversial and widely supported, focused on the issue of portability. The more partisan House bill contained a number of provisions that were likely to elicit a veto from President Clinton. The differences between the bills reflected the different natures of the two chambers. Speaker of the House Newt Gingrich used his substantial power to push a conservative agenda in the House. The Senate, however, is far more decentralized. Individual Senators can place holds on legislation and use the filibuster to effectively require sixty votes to end debate and pass a measure. The Senate also had more moderate Republican members than it does today. Back then, compromise was a real option.

THE SENATE

Senator Nancy Kassebaum (R-Kans.) and Senator Edward Kennedy (D-Mass.) were the chair and ranking member, respectively, of the Senate Committee on Health and Human Services, and their leadership made HIPAA possible. This law is often referred to as "the Kennedy Kassebaum bill," but it was actually the Kassebaum Kennedy bill.[5] The bill was passed unanimously by their committee (16-0) and ultimately secured a unanimous vote on the Senate floor (98-0). The bill had sixty-five co-sponsors, which Senator John Breaux (D-La.) referred to as a "large but fragile coalition." It took a complex balancing act to create consensus. Liberals in the Senate viewed HIPAA as a modest step toward more significant reform, moderates saw it as an issue of fairness, and conservatives saw it as a way to streamline rules and regulations. Senator Kennedy called HIPAA "a constructive step forward" and "a modest bill, an important bill."[6] Another liberal, Senator Jay Rockefeller (D-W.Va.), said that wide-scale reform would "have to wait for a renewed demand, a broader demand, a broader anger on the part of the American people."[7] Moderate Republican Senator Jim Jeffords (R-Vt.) said that the goal of the legislation was to "level the playing field in the self-funded ERISA market by applying the same national rules to both segments of the market place."[8] Senator Bill Roth (R-Del.), a conservative Republican, said that "there is a need to establish uniform standards for group-to-group portability measures, as the bulk of employer-sponsored health coverage is self-funded and exempt from state regulation."[9]

The Senate bill's core provisions aimed to make insurance products more widely available and automatically renewable. It also restricted coverage exclusions based on preexisting conditions: an important provision allowed insurance companies to exclude only conditions diagnosed and treated in the previous six months and to deny coverage for only a single year. Consider this hypothetical case: Leslie has been uninsured for the last year, and just last month she was diagnosed with a liver disease. If Leslie signs up for insurance, her liver treatments can still be excluded for a period of twelve months. But if Leslie had already had insurance for at least a year with no gaps in coverage longer than sixty-three days, her preexisting condition would have been covered immediately, even if she switched insurance. The complexity of the regulations arises from the fact that not everyone has coverage. Insurance companies do not want people waiting until they are sick to buy insurance, and they can make a lot of money by dropping coverage for sick people. That is why the individual coverage mandate included in the Patient Protection and Affordable Care Act is essential to truly eliminating preexisting condition exclusions.

The Senate bill moved the federal government into an area traditionally regulated by the states. In the case of HIPAA, legislators' stance on issues of federalism depended on context; attitudes toward the degree of federal or state control of health insurance regulations were directly related to immediate policy goals. For example, the late Senator Paul Wellstone (D-Minn.), perhaps the most liberal member of the Senate, argued for state control when he said that "states should be able to pass stronger consumer protection regulations and have them apply to all people in the state."[10] Traditionally, state preemption arguments come from conservatives. At the same time, Wellstone and other liberals argued for stronger national regulations to protect patients. For example, the left wing wanted to limit the ability of insurance plans to increase premiums for sicker or older beneficiaries. Legislators on both the left and right sought to allocate responsibility to the level of government most likely to forward their policy goals.

On the other end of the political spectrum, Senator Bob Dole (R-Kans.) introduced a number of amendments that would increase the power of the federal government to forward conservative goals. The most far-reaching provision was the creation of medical savings accounts (MSAs), which are tax-free savings accounts that work with high-deductible plans. If an employer offered a health plan with a $5,000 deductible, the employee could set up an account to which she and her employer could contribute $5,000 tax free to the MSA. The money in the account could be used only for health care–related payments. The MSA provision would have diminished state regulation and incorporated new federal standards that favored higher-income people with more to gain from the tax advantages and less to lose from higher out-of-pocket costs.[11] In contrast to what one might expect, national insurance regulation was advocated most strongly by the most conservative members of Congress.

Most discussions that were explicitly about federalism centered on state flexibility in the individual insurance market and the thorny issue of regulating costs. Republicans and Democrats both highlighted the importance of ensuring state flexibility to develop alternative mechanisms for people moving into the complex individual insurance market, which is characterized by tremendous variation among states with respect to insurance products, regulations, and programs. It is also very expensive because people shopping for individual insurance tend to be relatively older and more likely to need and use medical care. Many states subsidize individual insurance through high-risk pools, but HIPAA provided no subsidies. Therefore, in the interest of keeping the bill noncontroversial, federal legislators granted states considerable flexibility in regulating the individual insurance market.

Federal legislators deferred to the states on the issue of how much insurance companies would be allowed to charge. Even though insurance companies might no longer routinely exclude coverage for preexisting conditions, they could still exclude high-cost individuals and companies by pricing products out of their reach. In response to criticism that HIPAA did not regulate how much could be charged for premiums, Senator Kassebaum replied, "We do not preempt states from doing community rating [setting one mandatory rate for a state or community] or a cap, if a state so desires." She added that flexibility was one of the reasons that "we have the strong support of the state insurance commissioners and the National Governors

Association."[12] Though states had the power to set rate restrictions, their influence was limited to non-ERISA plans. Pacifying critics, Senator Jeffords noted that there were "much-needed improvements at the national level but at the same time [the bill] allows states the flexibility they need to move ahead in their own efforts."[13]

HIPAA was necessary because states did not have the authority to regulate insurance plans provided by large companies. Meanwhile, state actions were used to gain support to expand federal regulation. State flexibility was invoked to keep consensus and avoid the controversial step of regulating how much health insurance plans could charge different people and businesses. It was like a game of "hot potato." Both federal and state governments wanted to avoid upsetting the insurance industry, but each hoped that the other level of government would take responsibility. Federalism can enable consensus by keeping things ambiguous, but it can also turn into an intergovernmental shell game.

THE HOUSE OF REPRESENTATIVES

The House called its bill the Health Coverage Availability and Affordability Act of 1996, suggesting that it had far more ambitious goals than the insurance reform bill pushed by the Senate. The House bill was crafted by four committees: the Ways and Means Committee, the Committee on Economic and Educational Opportunities, the Commerce Committee, and the Judiciary Committee. The Commerce Committee drafted the insurance provisions, the Ways and Means Committee promoted MSAs, and the Judiciary Committee added provisions on medical malpractice. Throughout this process, the House leadership tightly controlled the bill. Amendments were not allowed, but Democrats were able to present an alternative, the Roukema-Kassebaum-Kennedy bill, which was identical to the Senate bill.[14]

The House Republican leadership viewed this legislation as the final stage of health care reform; it was the conservative version of national health care reform. Speaker Gingrich boasted that "we went . . . past portability to affordability."[15] He called the Senate version "well-meaning, but . . . inadequate. It is too little, it is too narrow, it is too small; we can do better." Dennis Hastert (R-Ill.), chief deputy whip and chairman of the Republican Health Care Taskforce, said, "Our legislation will lower the cost of health care insurance while making it more available and affordable to middle-income families."[16] Ways and Means Committee chairman Bill Archer (R-Tex.) observed that "after years of talking about health reform, we are now, with the new Republican majority in the House, going to enact health reform."[17] Despite those claims, there was little evidence that the House's approach would have covered the uninsured or significantly reduced health care costs. In opposition to any notion of devolution, accomplishing the goals of the House bill would have required increased federal authority over the states.

The House bill differed from the Senate's in several significant ways. The House bill included MSAs, which supporters argued would decrease the cost of insurance and increase access. It allowed small employers to join together in multiple employer work associations (MEWAs), which would make them exempt from state insurance regulation, just like the larger ERISA plans. That provision was justified by claims that state regulations added as much as 30 percent to the cost of insurance for a small business.[18] The House bill included caps on awards for medical malpractice claims, and it allowed tax deductions for the purchase of long-term care insurance (a plank in the Contract with America).[19] In addition, it doubled the length of time that people could go without health insurance and still enjoy protection from exclusions based on preexisting coverage.

Apart from the question of whether they would have achieved their stated goals, those proposals all shifted power from the states to the federal government, even though Republicans claimed that medical savings accounts would empower individuals and reduce aggregate government power. Jack Kingston (R-Ga.) said that MSAs gave Americans choices: "It takes it away from our Washington bureaucrat command and control allies and puts it in the hands of the American public where it belongs."[20] While MSAs may have provided greater options for certain individuals, they required an increase in federal regulation of insurance plans. MSAs would be set up under federal guidelines and national regulations preempting state law. For example, employers would be required by federal law to contribute to the MSAs of eligible employees or they would incur tax penalties. Further, the level of the annual deduction was set by the federal government, as was the definition of "medical expenditure." MSAs represented a clear expansion of federal jurisdiction over health insurance.

The same dynamic applied to MEWAs, which would enable small businesses to be exempted from state regulation. Speaker Gingrich justified federal intervention by saying that "large self-insured businesses are exempt from state law, in their health plans, while small business is stuck with state insurance coverage mandates, premium taxes, and other forms of regulation."[21] Harris Fawell (R-Ill.) viewed this as an issue of equity, stating that small businesses just wanted the same right to be "exempt from state laws" as large self-insured companies.[22] Republicans wanted to eliminate state regulation of small businesses and replace it with weaker federal standards.

Conservatives held to the notion that government power in Washington is bad, except when it forwards their interests. Ironically, federal power was enlisted to protect people and businesses against the state governments.

Democrats seized on the irony of Republican expansion of federal power. Bill Clay (D-Mo.) noted the historically high levels of fraud and abuse associated with MEWAs and pointed out that centralized regulation of those entities by the Department of Labor would be difficult and weak. Ben Cardin (D-Md.) declared, "We are trying to return power to the states. This bill moves in exactly the opposite direction. It preempts our states without providing adequate federal protection."[23] He added, "The net effect of the final provision relating to MEWAs is extremely damaging to state authority to govern their own insurance market. We are moving in the wrong direction by taking more power, rather than giving our states the ability to control health insurance."[24] The always quotable Barney Frank (D-Mass.) said, "This bill is the government increasing its role in health. . . . It is a great repudiation of their [Republicans'] own philosophy."[25] Peter DeFazio (D-Ore.) also noted that "ironically, H.R. 3103 [the House version of HIPAA] would also remove state oversight and replace it with federal regulations to advantage insurance companies. This would be a severe blow to the states' rights movement."[26]

The Republicans never responded directly to such criticism; for the most part, they stayed focused on their goals. However, they did show some willingness to compromise on the issue of individual coverage. Tom Bliley (R-Va.) and others said that states would be given the flexibility to "achieve individual coverage through a variety of means that include risk pools, group conversion policies, open enrollment by one or more insurers, and guaranteed issue."[27] The Republican leadership did not want to dictate the design of the individual market, "as long as they [the states] met some really broad criteria."[28]

With that exception, Republicans avoided a discussion of federalism altogether. The House bill was ambiguous about the states' ability to regulate insurance beyond HIPAA standards. The National Association of Insurance Commissioners (NAIC) and the National Conference of State Legislatures (NCSL) wrote a letter to Speaker Gingrich asking for greater state flexibility. The House bill stated that it did not preempt state laws that "relate to matters not specifically addressed in the bill," but those organizations wanted explicit language spelling out the states' authority to regulate ERISA plans. States also wanted to know how far they could move beyond HIPAA standards when regulating non-ERISA plans.[29] Ultimately, the organizations were disappointed that such language was never included. The conservative

Republican leadership and states' rights advocates were on opposite sides of this issue.

Although the House and Senate bills took different approaches, they both drove home the same lessons about federal and state relations. The Senate bill was crafted to attract widespread support; controversial issues were kept at bay by the sponsors' skillful maneuvering. The House bill attempted to go further by addressing issues of affordability. Conservatives in the Senate supported an increased role for the federal government, while some liberals supported the states' right to exceed federal standards. Both chambers provided state flexibility in the individual insurance market, where there was no consensus on federal action. Historically, this area had been regulated by the states. The more conservative House leadership forwarded policy to curb state regulation and expand the federal government's role. Parties pushed for power at the level of government that best promoted their policy objectives, often in contrast to their typical ideological stands on federalism.

ROLE OF THE STATES

The National Association of Insurance Commissioners, the National Conference of State Legislatures, and the National Governors Association (NGA) actively pushed for states' interests throughout the legislative process. The NAIC and NCSL provided technical assistance to members of Congress and their staffs and closely followed the progress of the legislation. Charles N. Kahn III, staff director of the House Ways and Means Committee at the time, said that the governors were not as engaged in HIPAA as in CHIP and that it was the state legislators (through NCSL) and the state insurance commissioners (through NAIC) who were engaged on the details of the bill.[30] That was entirely predictable. Governors are not directly involved in insurance on a day-to-day basis, largely because it does not have the direct budget impact of Medicaid and CHIP.[31] Dean Rosen (Senator Kassebaum's key staff person) pointed out that nevertheless, the governors were the most critical state actors and their support, opposition, or neutrality was of concern to HIPAA's sponsors.[32] In fact, Kennedy's and Kassebaum's staff worked through the NAIC to increase the governors' level of comfort and to obtain their eventual support.[33]

Congressional staff said that NAIC did not have much direct political influence in Congress because its constituency was so dispersed. They noted that NCSL's political influence also was weak because different state legislatures have such diverse interests.[34] Nevertheless, the insurance commissioners and, to a lesser degree, the state legislatures played an important role in the debate by providing technical information to members of Congress and their staffs. The commissioners' input was based on expertise and knowledge from states that wrote the existing laws and knew the potential pitfalls and loopholes. NAIC and NCSL were active in trying to get legislative committees to understand the impact of the legislation on states,[35] and both groups made the case that Congress should not undo the considerable work that the states had already done.[36] The states' advantage with respect to information and expertise about insurance regulation gave them power and influence, and that became a central theme of HIPAA rulemaking and implementation.

The information provided by NAIC, much of which was directed to the Senate, directly influenced the specifics of the legislation. An NAIC official noted that the relationship between Congress and the states was based on mutual need and reciprocity.[37] Senator Kassebaum's staff confirmed the cooperative nature of this relationship but pointed out that NAIC's influence was more technical than political.[38] Information on state programs helped congressional staff set a time frame for such things as allowable exclusion periods and acceptable gaps in coverage. Staff wanted to be in the same ballpark as the states. Senator Kassebaum's staff said that tables detailing state programs and timetables were extremely helpful in setting federal parameters.[39]

Moreover, state organizations collaborated with industry when state flexibility was in their mutual interest. In the same vein, the health insurance companies allied with governors to influence national policy.[40] For example, industry joined with the states in opposition to MEWA provisions for small businesses proposed in the House. Further, insurers that did not want to meet potentially expensive federal requirements in the individual insurance market joined with governors to support state authority and flexibility in this area. Ultimately, the collaboration of state organizations with the governors weakened federal requirements and increased state options. That strategy was successful in watering down the legislation as it worked its way through the House and Senate.[41]

With very different pieces of legislation coming out of the two chambers of Congress, a joint House-Senate conference committee was convened to hammer out the final version. Conference committee meetings were held behind closed doors.[42] What emerged was insurance reform that resembled the Senate version, with compromises on measures included in the House bill. The statute provided for an MSA demonstration program, a tax deduction for the self-employed, a long-term care insurance tax deduction, and federal standards for administrative simplification of insurance forms. It did not allow small business to join together to avoid state regulation.

GROUP MARKET

HIPAA states that portability provisions in the group market do not supersede state laws unless state laws attempt to prohibit the implementation of federal requirements. Generally, when states have higher standards and stronger requirements that do not conflict with HIPAA, state law prevails. But again, any stronger provisions will not be applied to ERISA-protected plans.[43] States do not have the flexibility to develop alternative approaches in the group insurance market, even if the approaches offer more protection than base federal standards. States must comply with federal preexisting condition provisions, although they can make particular provisions within the standard stronger. For example, the statute specifies seven areas in which the states can increase protection of consumers against the exclusion of coverage of preexisting conditions.[44]

States can increase consumer protection by shortening the exclusion period, broadening the definition of what counts as a preexisting condition and is therefore protected from coverage exclusion, or adding opportunities for special enrollment, but they cannot change the overall structure or framework of the program. This is circumscribed flexibility: states cannot implement an alternative approach, and they are not allowed to meet or better the standard however they want.[45] States still could not regulate ERISA plans, so any changes that they made would not apply to self-funded plans in their state. That was a win for both big business and labor. The impact was limited in other, less obvious ways. The statute mandated that newborns and adopted children cannot be excluded from coverage because of preexisting conditions and that pregnancy cannot be defined as a preexisting condition. These provisions sound important, but in practice they accomplished little because states already had such policies in place.[46]

States are still free to regulate premiums and benefits for non-ERISA plans, but most are reluctant to enact strong regulations affecting the powerful insurance industry. Even if they wanted to get tough, their influence could extend only so far. In the group market, HIPAA prohibits insurers from basing eligibility for and renewability of insurance on health status, current medical conditions, past health care claims, medical history, genetic information, and evidence of insurability or disability. However, nothing in this law prohibits insurance companies from changing benefits and/or increasing premiums at the end of a contract period. So while the insurance carrier may no longer drop coverage for a small business that, for example, has an employee diagnosed with cancer, they can raise the firm's rate so high that renewal is impossible. That is especially harmful for individuals and small businesses, since large companies can spread the cost of one very sick employee across a large number of employees. While some states regulated this practice, most did not, thus limiting the effectiveness of HIPAA. That disparity drove President Obama and congressional Democrats to seek additional protection under ACA. New health exchanges hold the possibility of combining small businesses together in the same insurance pool to protect them from major premium hikes associated with one employee who has an expensive illness.

INDIVIDUAL MARKET

States have greater flexibility in the individual market than in the group market. HIPAA guarantees renewability in this market and protects people with preexisting conditions. People moving from the group to the individual market can avoid the preexisting condition exclusion if they have twelve months of previous coverage with no breaks longer than sixty-three days. These specific provisions do not apply if a state develops an "acceptable alternative mechanism" approved by the federal government.[47] Alternative mechanisms must also meet certain requirements, but the statute proactively approves initiatives already in place in many states. At a minimum, the state must provide individuals a choice of several comprehensive coverage plans. A number of public and private mechanisms were given as examples of acceptable options for the states, including the kind of risk pool arrangements already in place in many states. While group market regulations require a specific program but give states flexibility to change details, the individual market regulations present federal goals and allow states greater flexibility in determining how they are achieved.

ENFORCEMENT

The law sets monetary penalties for noncompliant insurers,[48] but regulating the actions of states, which have constitutionally protected powers, is far more complex. The courts have said that the federal government cannot simply require states to do its administrative bidding. For comparison, the federal government can set state standards for programs such as CHIP and Medicaid because states are not required to have either program. But if they opt out, they will miss out on federal funding. Courts have consistently ruled that the federal government can essentially buy compliance by threatening to withhold funds. For example, when the federal government wanted the states to increase the drinking age to 21 years, it could not just issue a decree.

Instead, it said that only states that adopted the standard would be eligible for federal highway funding. Is it surprising that every state complied?

HIPAA is different because it does not provide states with significant funding. With HIPAA, the penalty for noncompliance is that the federal government will come in and enforce the rules. That gave the states the option of not operating a program and having the federal government come in and do it instead. States could also pick and choose which provisions they wanted to adopt and shift enforcement responsibilities to the federal government for provisions that they chose not to enact. That turned out not to be an intergovernmental strategy designed for success.

During the legislative process, federal legislators, staff, and interest groups assumed that no state would invite federal regulators to take over insurance regulation in their state. They assumed that the very threat of federal interference would compel states to stick closely to the rules. They could not have been more wrong. The rulemaking and implementation chapters show that the federal government, like an absentee landlord, abdicated oversight responsibility, and the law fell into disrepair. Similarly, under ACA, the state penalty for not setting up a health exchange is that the federal government will step in and take over. If HIPAA is any indication, however, this enforcement mechanism may not work out as planned.

During consideration of HIPAA, conservatives abandoned ideological notions of federalism to support overriding policy goals. They wanted to decrease overall government power by exempting a larger number of businesses from state regulation and subjecting them to weaker federal rules. They also wanted to increase individual control of health care through medical savings accounts and tax deductions for long-term care insurance. Each of those objectives increased federal authority and ran counter to the notion of devolution of federal power to the states. But even while Democrats cried hypocrisy, some liberals advocated for states' rights—and against their usual ideological leaning—to give consumers more aggressive protections.

The rhetoric of federalism was prominent during the creation of CHIP but conspicuously absent in much of the HIPAA debate. In both cases policy was foreshadowed in the states and paved the way for federal action. In both cases federalism was used less as an ideology and more as a political tool to support or defeat particular policy goals. States influenced the development of HIPAA and CHIP, but the sources of influence and the actors were different in each case. The governors were more active in CHIP and worked directly with members of Congress. NAIC and NCSL played a more direct role in drafting the details of HIPAA and worked more at the staff level. Neither political party was willing to give the states authority over the issues that they cared most deeply about. With HIPAA, both parties deferred to the states when it came time to regulate premiums, which is essential for providing individuals and small business with true protection against catastrophic costs. Here federalism was used to avoid responsibility and shift power to another level of government or to the regulated community.

Evidence from CHIP and HIPAA indicates that in a conservative era, the best chance of forwarding progressive legislation may be to build on policy at the state level. CHIP, HIPAA, and the Massachusetts health care reform are all examples of state policy influencing national developments. It is already clear that state policies also are playing a central role in the implementation of national reform.

HIPAA legislation made progress toward reducing the preexisting conditions exclusion. Successful implementation offered the real possibility that people with heart disease, diabetes, or other medical conditions would be covered when they changed employers and therefore insurance plans. The failure to regulate costs, however, weakened those provisions. The real impact of the program could not be known until the rules were specified by administrative agencies and programs were actually implemented in the states. It is to these details that I now turn.

CHAPTER SIX

HIPAA:
FEDERALISM AND RULEMAKING

The rulemaking process that turned HIPAA legislation into policy should serve as a cautionary tale for national reform through the Patient Protection and Affordable Care Act. The HIPAA rule used the threat of a federal takeover of a state regulatory function to enforce the insurance portability provisions. However, because the federal government did not have the resources, staff, expertise, or desire to back up the threat, it capitulated to the states during the rulemaking process, thereby weakening the law. Similarly, if the states refuse to create health care exchanges under the ACA, the only recourse is for the federal government to step in and run the exchanges.

Indeed, the federal government seemed to follow this pattern in drafting the early ACA rules governing health care exchanges, bending over backward to cajole the states into participating by designing weak and flexible rules.[1] This approach weakens federal efforts to achieve uniformity, but it may increase state engagement, which is critical for success. The federal government is in a difficult position with respect to the ACA, in contrast to its experience with CHIP, when it was dealing from a position of strength. With CHIP it had the expertise, resources, and staff—along with financial incentives and penalties—to compel the states to act and to work with them to achieve program goals.

HIPAA was signed into law on August 21, 1996. As with CHIP, Congress wanted the program up and running as quickly as possible. The Centers for Medicare and Medicaid Services (CMS), the Department of Labor Pension and Welfare Benefits Administration (PWBA), and the Department of the Treasury issued joint regulations to speed up the process. As with CHIP, federal-state relations helped shape the HIPAA rule. This time, however, the states ended up dominating the rulemaking process; in fact, they literally wrote large sections of the law.

Many factors contributed to the near-collapse of federal authority over the HIPAA rulemaking process. In the end, the feds were sunk by overly ambitious deadlines, dispersed rulemaking responsibilities, limited federal expertise, staff and resource shortfalls, and lack of state reporting requirements or any other way to hold states and insurance companies accountable. Conversely, states gained leverage through their historical expertise in regulating insurance. It is not surprising, when one looks back, that any ambiguity in the law was settled in favor of the states. While the law reads like federal encroachment on state responsibility, the rulemaking process revealed a toothless federal government. On one hand, given diverse state insurance markets and the ambiguity regarding what an efficient exchange looks like, considerable flexibility might be a good thing. On the other, "anything goes" exchanges could lead to news exposés about inefficient exchanges that waste taxpayers' money, reducing the credibility of reform.

TIME FRAME

HIPAA was passed with remarkably ambitious timelines. According to the legislation, health plans and health insurance carriers had to comply with the new law just one year after passage, but before that could happen, each state had to enact new laws to make compliance possible. For states with legislatures that meet only once or twice a year, the schedule was unrealistic.[2] States wanting to create alternative programs in the individual insurance market had to submit a letter of intent within the first eight months, even before federal guidance outlining program parameters was issued.[3] Furthermore, less than a year after passage, health issuers were required to issue certificates to employees documenting continuous coverage. That required making changes in information technology systems before the federal or state governments issued any guidelines—a risky proposition since much can be invested in vain if requirements change, as they often do.

Issuance of federal HIPAA insurance regulations was fast-tracked in a manner known as "interim and final." It sounds like a contradiction in terms, but that's just business as usual. Rules are usually released first as "a notice of proposed rulemaking" to give interested parties the opportunity to comment; this first release requires a response from federal agencies. In contrast, interim and final rules have the immediate force of law, and Congress had authorized issuing the rules as final if a longer comment period would be "impracticable."[4] Because of the tight deadlines, the federal government pledged not to take enforcement action until after January 1, 1998, if states' plans and employers were making a "good-faith effort" to comply.

AGENCY REGULATIONS

Regulations were issued jointly by CMS, PWBA, and the Treasury Department. CMS was responsible for drafting rules and regulations for the individual and group insurance markets that guaranteed portability; the rules were to be concurrent with state responsibilities, and CMS hoped that state enforcement would be the norm. PWBA was responsible for enforcing amendments that apply to employers and to large companies that self-insure (ERISA plans). Treasury was responsible for enforcing HIPAA amendments to the tax code, but it did not have sole jurisdiction over any particular aspect of the law or rule. An interagency work group was established to coordinate writing of the group market regulations. Drafts were circulated and issues were resolved before submission to the Office of Management and Budget (OMB) for clearance. This process represents how the federal bureaucracy works.

CENTERS FOR MEDICARE AND MEDICAID SERVICES

CMS's jurisdiction in the group and individual markets made it a central player in the rulemaking process. CMS had limited experience in the direct regulation of insurance companies, and initially it had no funds for HIPAA oversight.[5] CMS's first experience regulating Medicare supplemental (Medigap) policies in the 1980s foreshadowed its HIPAA experience. Medigap policies provide wraparound coverage for the Medicare program, which obliges participants to pay considerable out-of-pocket costs. States traditionally regulated Medigap products, but because there was concern at the national level that state oversight left room for widespread fraud, CMS was tasked with certifying that Medigap plans met certain standards. During that process, the National Association of Insurance Commissioners (NAIC) wrote draft standards, which eventually were codified by CMS. States meeting the NAIC standards retained control of their Medigap markets. In the end, all states adopted those standards, so CMS never developed the staff expertise or administrative capacity to certify any plans or state policies. The Medigap experience did not prepare CMS to regulate private insurance, and neither would HIPAA. Not surprisingly, current efforts to draft ACA insurance regulations are confronting similar limits with respect to federal expertise and administrative capacity to regulate insurance.

State governments had more tools to enforce HIPAA regulations than the federal government did. The feds made it clear in the preamble to the HIPAA rules that states have primary responsibility for enforcing HIPAA provisions in the group and individual market, except with respect to self-insured ERISA plans. The group health plan regulation reads, "Only if a State does not substantially enforce any provisions under its insurance law will the Department of Health and Human Services [through CMS] enforce the provisions, through the imposition of civil money penalties."[6] CMS could impose civil penalties on health plans or insurers of up to $100 per violation per day. But the states have the real power here. They have various options to enforce compliance, including "criminal and civil penalties, cease and desist orders, injunctions, removal of officers and directors and revocation or refusal to renew licenses."[7] Few people believed that CMS would ever have to take over state regulatory functions. In fact, the regulations explicitly stated, "It is highly unlikely that there will be any instances of the federal government assuming such a role, with the exception perhaps of the territories."[8]

CMS administrator Bruce Vladeck made it clear at congressional hearings that his agency would defer to the states.[9] Still, Senator Mike Enzi (R-Wyo.) feared that CMS would be quick to assert control over the states. He was especially concerned about how CMS would define state "good-faith efforts." But there was never any need for concern; Vladeck said that "any effort" would be considered a good-faith effort and that the federal government would do everything possible to avoid a takeover.[10] Later, Senator Enzi asked Joy Wilson, the National Conference of State Legislatures (NCSL) representative, if her members had any concerns about federal agencies going beyond the standards in the law. She replied, "I think that the federal agencies are basically urging us to come into compliance. I do not think they want to regulate these laws in the states any more than we want them to."[11] This approach is a stark contrast to the way that states were treated during the formal CHIP rulemaking process.

STATE INFLUENCE

Despite the fast-tracking of the regulations, the states played a significant role in their development. CMS established a symbiotic relationship with the states, largely through the state insurance commissioners, represented by NAIC. At times, NAIC wrote large portions of the rule. NAIC provided the states with the model laws and regulations necessary to implement HIPAA's provisions;[12] it even developed the state implementation manual. State representatives could not have been more pleased. Joy Wilson, speaking for NCSL, said that "CMS has been as helpful as they can be."[13] Josephine Musser, president of the NAIC, said that the federal agencies and the states shared the same goal, which was "for the states to succeed."[14] Indeed, federal officials were in constant contact with NAIC, attended its quarterly meetings, and relied heavily on its data. The General Accounting Office's first-year assessment of HIPAA concluded that "states and the insurance industry were generally pleased with the open and inclusive nature of the [rulemaking] process."[15] All of that should have added up to a big red flag: when the regulated are so demonstrably pleased, the strength of the regulations should be seriously doubted.

The relationship that CMS had with the states in implementing HIPAA differed from the relationship that they had in implementing Medicaid and CHIP. States were not required to submit detailed program information about their compliance with HIPAA.[16] Bruce Vladeck, the CMS administrator at the time, explained that "states are not required to send us their updated group laws or regulations, and we have no authority, on the group side, to approve or disapprove them."[17] In fact, House and Senate conferees rejected a Senate provision that would have required the states to develop and file enforcement plans with CMS.[18] The CMS administrator said that responsibility for enforcement action should rest with the states, which "have the depth of experience necessary to successfully fill this role."[19] A former national director of state Medicaid directors said that CMS had a more collaborative relationship with the states with HIPAA than with CHIP and speculated that that may have been because HIPAA "wasn't part of their core mission. Their passion and energy were not directed there."[20] CMS also had to deal with inadequate resources, inexperienced staff, an insufficient knowledge base, and lack of the infrastructure necessary to regulate thousands of insurance carriers in diverse local markets.

INDUSTRY AND CONSUMER GROUPS

Just like politicians, industry and consumer groups wanted power to go to whichever level of government best advanced their goals. Through comments on the rule, congressional testimony, and my interviews with senior Health Insurance Association of America (HIAA) staff, it became clear that the insurance industry did not object to (and may even benefit from) some uniform national insurance standards. At the same time, the industry was more comfortable with state than with federal enforcement of HIPAA. Consumer groups wanted to make sure that HIPAA regulations did not turn into a ceiling that prevented states from exceeding federal requirements;

they also wanted to prevent the rollback of more protective state laws that were already in existence. Moreover, consumer groups wanted strong federal oversight of some of the state insurance commissioners, who at times seemed to be captives of the industry.

The industry found itself in the odd position of advocating for federal regulation. An industry representative testified before a congressional oversight hearing that HIPAA regulations should "reinforce the primacy of federal standards and limit future state action."[21] An official at HIAA confirmed that uniform national standards can be more beneficial than a wide range of decentralized requirements.[22] However, HIAA stressed that states have primary enforcement powers and that federal action may take place only when the state fails to "substantially enforce" the law. They wanted the best of both worlds.

Meanwhile, the insurance industry already enjoyed a cozy relationship with many states. Through the NAIC, the state insurance commissioners worked closely with HIAA and largely shared its view on enforcement. Josephine Musser, the NAIC president, stated that "the act allows each state the flexibility to adopt whatever sanctions or remedy it believes necessary to carry out the provisions of the legislation."[23]

Gail Shearer of the Consumers Union testified that the insurance industry wielded great power in many states. In fact, she warned, the industry intended to use HIPAA to eliminate consumer protections that exceeded the federal minimums and consumer groups were afraid that "HIPAA could in fact become a ceiling." She told Congress that "we [the Consumers Union] do not believe that Congress intended that HIPAA be an excuse for industry to strong-arm states into rolling back established state policies that go further than the minimums in HIPAA."[24]

The industry wanted minimum uniform national standards enforced by states, and consumer groups wanted federal action to prevent the rollback of enhanced protections in the states. Industry largely prevailed. State discretion with national reform may similarly risk empowering the insurance industry and weakening national standards.

State Flexibility and Federal Control

The CHIP and HIPAA rules both stressed commitment to state flexibility. However, while the CHIP rule curtailed state discretion at every turn, the HIPAA rule deferred to the states at every opportunity. The rule reads that CMS "narrowly interpreted the preemption of state law [and thereby] provided states considerable flexibility in complying with the statute, and recognized the limited authority of federal agencies in the regulation of health insurance."[25] It further declares the goals of "preserving . . . the states' traditional role in regulating health insurance, including state flexibility to provide greater protections."[26] This is all bureaucratic speak suggesting that CMS would bend over backward to accommodate states. Where the law is clear and direct regarding federal government responsibilities, the rule follows suit, but whenever possible CMS wanted the states to retain as much of their traditional power to regulate health insurance as possible.

The Group Market

The group market rule is clear on federal-state relations. Federal standards are required, but states have considerable latitude to define specific parameters. States can change particular time frames or definitions to add protection, but they must use the general federal framework. Limits on preexisting condition exclusions, including acceptable gaps in coverage and look-back periods (periods for which people had previous continuous coverage), mirror those in the statute. The federal definition of "preexisting condition" preempts state law, and states with less protective policies are required to strengthen their standards. The rule defines a preexisting condition as a condition for which a diagnosis, advice, care, or treatment has been received from a licensed health care professional or for which a licensed health care professional has recommended treatment, whether the condition was treated or not. Some states use a more expansive, less protective definition based on any condition that a prudent layperson would have sought care for.[27] These sound like a pretty tough federal requirements, but the rules describing federal enforcement would render compliance with them close to optional.[28]

Some states argued that the guaranteed issue provision for small businesses (those having two to fifty employees) could be read as guaranteeing the availability of only a basic, standard plan. But federal officials did not agree and held firm, insisting that the law requires all products in a market to be available to all small businesses.[29] The rule noted that forty-one states had a small group market guaranteed issue provision prior to HIPAA. And although HIPAA and twenty-one of those states defined "small group" differently,[30] it was predicted that only small changes would be necessary to comply with federal standards.[31] So, even where the regulations clearly specified federal authority, the rule went out of its way to explain that states would not have a problem with implementation. Again, in contrast, the implementation challenges that the states might face were never mentioned in the CHIP rule.

Insurers were also required to renew plans, with exceptions for nonpayment, fraud, and abuse. Plans were still allowed to modify benefits and coverage terms at the time of renewal "provided modification is consistent with state law, and for the small group market, is effectively uniform among group health plans with coverage under that product."[32] That means that unless prohibited by state law, an insurance company at annual renewal could, for example, drop dialysis coverage for a bakery whose chef was just diagnosed with kidney failure. Further, unless regulated by the state, plans could still increase premiums or add copayments and deductibles, which could effectively make insurance unaffordable and therefore unavailable.

Unlike with CHIP, federal agencies were cognizant of the potential burden that HIPAA posed to states. As if to ease their collective conscience—or at least to head off complaints—they pointed out existing state programs as evidence that compliance with regulations would not be onerous. For example, the rule reads that "all but two states had enacted some type of small group market reform, and 35 states had enacted some type of individual insurance reform."[33] Before HIPAA, thirty-seven states required guaranteed availability of at least some plans in the small group market, and forty-three states required guaranteed renewability.[34] The rule goes to great lengths to document that the majority of existing state regulations already met that requirement. Regulators quoted Congressional Budget Office estimates that the impact of state enforcement of the provisions would be "marginal."[35] Where the law was clear, the rule followed suit and was not influenced by state concerns. However, once again federal officials highlighted the minimal impact that the rule would have on the states.

PORTABILITY FROM THE GROUP TO THE INDIVIDUAL MARKET

States gained more flexibility in the individual market, where they were allowed to implement alternative mechanisms. CMS stated that "the individual health insurance market provisions of HIPAA recognize that States play the primary role in the regulation of insurance" and that it would "afford the States great flexibility in implementing the reforms required by the statute."[36] The rule noted that thirty-five states had already enacted some type of individual insurance reform and that thirty states were expected to implement alternative mechanisms. It cited a RAND study that reported that forty-two states had guaranteed issue rules in the individual market or a high-risk pool that could qualify as an acceptable alternative mechanism.[37] HIPAA required that all individual health insurance coverage be guaranteed to be renewable. If a state elected to use an alternative mechanism to guarantee availability, it still had to enforce the guaranteed renewability provision.

States had several options: they could develop or modify alternative mechanisms to meet federal standards for access to individual health coverage; they could adopt and administer federal "fallback" standards; or they could do nothing and have federal officials enforce the federal fallback position. Each option provided significant state flexibility. CMS had ninety days after a state's submission of an alternative mechanism to act on it; if CMS did not act, the alternative was automatically allowed. If the alternative was disapproved, the state had an opportunity to amend it. Any significant changes had to be submitted to CMS for review 120 days before the change could be made.[38] Unlike with CHIP, Medicare, and Medicaid, the federal government was bending over backward to accommodate the states in implementing HIPAA.

The federal fallback standards also gave states some power to plot their own course. If a state chose this option, individual coverage had to be available—with no exceptions for preexisting conditions—to people who had eighteen months of previous coverage with no gaps longer than sixty-three days. States had the flexibility to limit plan availability to two policy forms. The definition of "policy forms" in the statute was left ambiguous, and CMS decided to leave the interpretation up to states. States still had to provide a choice of plans and could require issuers either to make all products available or, at a minimum, to offer their two most popular or representative policies. Again, there were no direct federal restrictions on the price of premiums.[39] States could change any of the requirements to make the program easier for individuals to qualify but not to make it more difficult.

The third option—having federal officials take responsibility for enforcing the federal fallback standards—provided the least state autonomy. The federal government would determine what constitutes a policy form and what options were available to individuals. This alternative does provide the states with an exit option. States can do nothing, and its citizens can still obtain the benefits of the program. In comparison, states can chose not to have a Medicaid or a CHIP program, but the federal government will not come in and run the program for them. If a state does not want to regulate an industry, the prospect of federal regulations may not be completely unwelcome. If a parent asks a child to clean his room, parental authority is not strengthened by threatening "or else I'll do it for you."

ENFORCEMENT

The rule on enforcement gave the impression that the federal government was serious. It reads that "state law cannot differ in any way from the federal requirements except to expand the protections in one of several ways specifically permitted by the statute."[40] However, the enforcement rule later makes it clear that CMS would make significant accommodations for the states and go to great lengths to avoid federal enforcement. The details of the rule showed that enforcement was set up to be reactive and conciliatory.

Specifically, states were given every opportunity to "exhaust any state remedies," thus making federal enforcement unnecessary.[41] The regulations outlined the procedures that would take place prior to a federal takeover: the first step would be to explore every possible state remedy; the second would be to continue informal and formal contact with key state officials and then to notify them of alleged state violations and the consequences.[42] Any deadlines would not take effect until all avenues had been tried. Even after initial notification, there remained an opportunity to extend the thirty-day period for "good cause." At that point, CMS could either approve the state's response, permit a reasonable period for the state to demonstrate evidence of state enforcement, or notify the state of its failure to substantially enforce provisions. Those procedures gave states opportunity upon opportunity to comply, in keeping with previous indications that CMS did not have the resources, experience, or desire to enforce HIPAA's provisions.

STATE REACTION

The NAIC suggested a number of changes to the rules. Surprisingly, most of their recommendations called for stronger federal standards. The state insurance commissioners were concerned that nothing in the rule prohibited health insurers from changing their benefits. Some states still had plans that excluded conditions such as pregnancy, diabetes, and hernias.[43] NAIC wanted national rules to stop health plans from changing benefits to effectively circumvent HIPAA's protection against pre-existing condition exclusions. Further, NAIC wanted CMS to require insurers to provide "a premium quote within a specific time, such as seven days or five working days." In the group market, that would prevent plans from forcing individuals to exceed the allowable sixty-three-day break in coverage. The NAIC was using its expertise and experience with similar regulations to alert federal officials to the ways in which insurers could evade the regulations.

However, on a number of issues, NAIC echoed industry concerns. For example, the NAIC wanted to prevent people with high-deductible plans (like a medical spending account plan) from switching to a more generous coverage plan (like an HMO plan) when they became sick. The NAIC said that "allowing states maximum flexibility to design their own rules with respect to this category would be the best way to recognize the unique nature of each state's health insurance market."[44] In summary, the NAIC's comments pushed for stronger federal standards, although the NAIC also wanted the states to retain some flexibility in implementation and enforcement.

HIPAA became a reality through an unusually symbiotic relationship between federal agencies and the states. The two sides shared a common goal: preventing direct federal intervention. The NAIC played a direct role on behalf of the states in developing HIPAA insurance rules. Industry and consumer groups favored the level of government that they believed would protect their interests best. Industry wanted minimum uniform national standards but favored state enforcement; consumer groups wanted to protect state efforts that went beyond federal minimums to prevent any backsliding on benefits.

Federalism, often seen as a tool of power and authority, can also be seen as a force for abdication. In the case of HIPAA, states wanted strong federal regulations and the feds wanted to leave the "dirty work" to the states. CMS did not want to take over state programs. The insurance industry largely supported HIPAA, and the rulemaking process certainly did not do much to threaten its support.

How aggressive will the federal government or the states be when the time comes to regulate insurance products through the new health exchanges? Sometimes federalism can be used as a shell game to avoid the political pain of regulating a powerful industry. HIPAA demonstrates the complexity of intergovernmental relations and the influence of an industry at different levels of government. Here industry got most of what it wanted: weak national regulations, state enforcement, and no national prohibitions against changing benefit packages or premiums.

The federal government needed the states to participate in and implement HIPAA willingly, and its dependence on them gave the states leverage. The states had the expertise, resources, and infrastructure necessary to regulate insurance; federal officials did not. The prospect of a federal takeover scared federal officials more than state officials. In contrast, CMS had the resources, experience, knowledge, history, and desire to enact CHIP. CMS had leverage over the states: it could withhold funds and its approval was necessary before modifications could be made. Furthermore, the CHIP rule included major reporting requirements.

Reporting requirements were essential to federal control. The requirements provided information not only to CMS but also to the advocacy community, the media, and researchers, and the information provided gave significant power to federal officials and helped promote national goals. HIPAA rules included few reporting requirements; they simply required that states provide information on their alternative mechanism in the individual market. States did not have to prove that state law conformed to federal requirements or to submit annual reports on their efforts in the individual or group market. It is difficult for the federal government to regulate something blind, especially if it wants to look the other way.

CMS administrators did not have ready-made administrative structures to tap into, and they did not have the resources, expertise, or detailed information about state programs to compel state action. The federal government did not have incentives to entice the states, nor did it have a big enough stick to force the states to comply with federal wishes. Further, insurance regulation was not part of the core function of the agencies responsible for rulemaking and oversight.

As part of national reform, states are required to create health exchanges to encourage competition between health plans. As with HIPAA, the federal government will depend on the states for implementation, and once again its dependence empowers the states. Federal rules will help guide the level of state flexibility, which in turn will shape the program. Under the threat of federal takeover, the states must have exchanges up and running by 2014, but they must demonstrate progress by 2013. And, as with HIPAA, the federal government still does not have the resources or expertise to take over insurance regulation in diverse state marketplaces. As the HIPPA analysis might predict, early federal rulemaking and guidance have been exceedingly deferential to the states. Specifically, federal officials pushed back the original 2012 deadlines to the end of 2013, implemented halfway measures creating a federal-state hybrid exchange that will eventually transition to a fully state-run exchange, and considered state provision plans as "good enough" for them to move forward.[45] Karen Ignani, CEO of America's Health Insurance Plan (AHIP), said that "this rule recognizes that states are in the best position to establish exchanges because they have the experience and local-market knowledge needed to best meet consumers' needs."[46]

The lessons of CHIP suggest a middle ground and potential path forward for national reform. CHIP provided state flexibility within federally defined corridors. States were kept in bounds through economic incentives (carrots) and enforcement mechanisms (sticks). In setting up health care exchanges, that might mean, for example, tying federal requirements for establishing state health care exchanges to the provision or withholding of federal tax subsidies. State reporting requirements also would be established and tied to state subsidies. Alternatively, the threat of federal takeover needs to be real, and the consequences need to be painful enough to ensure that states actually engage in the process.

But ultimately, the expertise and ability to regulate insurance resides in the states; the federal government, at least in the short term, is unlikely to develop the state-specific expertise necessary to do so. That makes it essential for the states to be part of a collaborative process, but engaging the states to integrate health care exchanges into their existing health care systems will require incentives and flexibility. Early rules show the federal government being deferential to states to encourage them to develop exchanges; however, either federal or state abdication weakens the possibility for successful implementation of this important aspect of national reform. With the ACA as with HIPAA, how programs impact people is determined by their implementation, to which I turn next.

CHAPTER SEVEN

HIPAA:
FEDERALISM AND
IMPLEMENTATION

As HIPAA became the law of the land, the federal government continued to defer to the states in important ways. Because of passive federal oversight, states took control of the scope and shape of insurance reforms, particularly in the individual market. In contrast to the implementation of the CHIP rule, which resulted in greater uniformity between states, implementation of HIPAA maintained the diversity that already existed among the states. Oversight was so weak that states could basically enact what they wanted, when they wanted. As a result, HIPAA largely failed to make insurance more available and affordable.[1] Implementation of the Patient Protection and Affordable Care Act requires early cooperation with the states and considerable flexibility, as did implementation of CHIP. However, if the federal government takes an approach to ACA similar to the one that it took with HIPAA—if it chooses to be extremely deferential to the states at every turn—national reform will surely meet with disaster.

The standoffish position of the federal government that was so evident during HIPAA rulemaking was even more pronounced during implementation. The federal government had no real leverage to make states comply. Even when states wanted intervention, the federal government was reluctant and slow to act. The lack of a requirement that the states report to the Centers for Medicare and Medicaid Services in fact rendered the federal government blind. Further, when Congress finally enacted funds for federal oversight, CMS chose to hire temporary contractors instead of building the institutional capacity for a long-term commitment to program oversight. The contrast in responsibilities, particularly between the Department of Labor and CMS, offers insight into the importance of institutional capacity, expertise, agency routines, reporting requirements, and resources. The implementation of HIPAA underscores the need for reporting requirements, real enforcement, and overall accountability as national reform is implemented.

STATE AND FEDERAL AGENCY ACTION

The three federal agencies responsible for HIPAA implementation—the Internal Revenue Service, the Department of Labor, and CMS—had different roles in the process and different relationships with the states. The Internal Revenue Service (IRS) had limited responsibility but a lot of clout. Any threat of action by the IRS certainly would have grabbed the attention of large businesses. The Department of Labor (DOL), through the Pension and Welfare Benefits Agency (PWBA), had more direct responsibility for implementation and oversight. Building on existing networks with employers, it established a collegial working relationship with the states. CMS was given a new set of responsibilities, but it had neither the expertise nor the resources to accomplish the task.

INTERNAL REVENUE SERVICE

The main job of the IRS, in coordination with DOL and CMS, was to impose tax penalties for noncompliance, but the agency took very little action during the implementation process. The IRS could have imposed an excise tax on employers that did not comply with HIPAA standards. For example, it could have penalized employers whose health plans failed to issue certificates in a timely manner. But that was never a priority. In 2003 the IRS was reorganized into four components, and at the time it was still unclear which unit or units would take the lead in HIPAA enforcement. A senior IRS official said that in general, enforcement was decentralized to agents who, with an understanding of HIPAA provisions, could take action against an employer health plan. However, there is no evidence that that was taking place.[2] DOL or CMS also had the authority to use the threat of IRS referral in the course of performing their oversight or implementation functions. There is no evidence that the agencies referred any plans to the IRS during that period, but the threat of potential IRS action could still have served as an additional incentive to comply. In any case, senior IRS officials had no reason to believe that any IRS enforcement action had ever been taken.

DEPARTMENT OF LABOR

The Pension and Welfare Benefits Agency of the Department of Labor was responsible for the oversight of employer benefit plans and had sole responsibility for HIPAA implementation by companies that self-insured under ERISA. Implementation and oversight were conducted largely through PWBA's regional offices, at the direction of the central office. DOL increased customer support staff and educated personnel about HIPAA issues. DOL reported that all of its staff were "trained to deal with both pension and health-related issues." DOL also developed HIPAA compliance steps and added them to guidelines for investigating employers and for regular reviews.[3]

The PWBA made an effort to inform employers and certain employees of their rights and responsibilities under HIPAA. In 1997, it gave presentations in ten cities and hosted forty additional presentations to employer groups, health plans, and state and local officials; it also simulcast one of its presentations to an additional seventy locations. The agency ran public service announcements and published and distributed 200,000 booklets on HIPAA and related federal laws, and it also maintained a website that provided detailed information for employers and employees. The PWBA worked with the National Association of Insurance Commissioners (NAIC) and exchanged lists of contacts to better direct consumer or employer complaints to the proper officials.

For the most part, the word got out. The General Accounting Office (GAO), NAIC, and others concluded that larger employers had a good understanding of the law and generally were in compliance with it. They also indicated that smaller employers and consumers had relatively little understanding of HIPAA protections and that in many instances, the information that they had was wrong. DOL field officials reported to the GAO that they were especially concerned about small businesses that self-funded their health plans and did not go through a third-party administrator. DOL suggested that smaller employers were more likely to be out of compliance than larger employers.[4]

DOL was in a much better position than CMS to assume its responsibilities. HIPAA expanded DOL's oversight role but restricted the department's responsibilities to its traditional clientele, employers whose employee benefit and pension plans were regulated under ERISA. The scope and nature of the regulations expanded, but not the regulated community. In contrast to CMS, the DOL had established systems and procedures that it could tap to provide information and to monitor requirements. It also established a working relationship with the states to help separate their responsibilities and steer employers and consumers to the proper official. PWBA knew what needed to be done and developed long- and short-term strategies for meeting those needs. Although that represented an increase in responsibility without a commensurate increase in resources, the task was not onerous. Most large firms were already in compliance, and enforcement action on smaller firms was taken only in the rare instances in which issues were brought to the DOL's attention.

The Centers for Medicare and Medicaid Services

HIPAA was a new responsibility for CMS, one that was outside the agency's core mission. In addition to working with the states and approving state alternative mechanisms in the individual market, CMS was responsible for the implementation of certain provisions in five states that were known to be out of compliance.[5] The agency was also tasked with taking enforcement action in any other state that failed to "substantially enforce" a portion of HIPAA. All states had some insurance reform regulations prior to HIPAA, some stronger than federal law and some weaker. If a state law did not conform to federal law, CMS was responsible for regulating the gaps between state law and HIPAA requirements. GAO concluded that "this created a complicated [and confusing] array of oversight for consumers, employers, and carriers of health coverage."[6]

For example, assume that a state defined "small employer" as any business with three to forty full-time employees. That state would be out of compliance with HIPAA, which defines small employers as having between two and fifty full- and part-time employees in total. If the state remained noncompliant, CMS would be responsible for enforcing HIPAA requirements for companies with two employees and those with between forty and fifty employees. That would require a double set of bureaucratic oversight procedures to accomplish essentially the same thing. To make things even more complicated, it was entirely possible that state and federal regulators could count part-time employees differently. Since base regulations and health insurance markets differ by state, the number of potential combinations of variables is immense. If that seemed complex and confusing, CMS was right there to help: it hoped to avoid setting up duplicative systems by just letting the states handle enforcement.

CMS had many other responsibilities, including responding to consumer inquiries and complaints, providing guidance to insurance carriers, imposing civil penalties for noncompliance, and reviewing carrier forms, policies, and practices.[7] Those tasks and more were already being performed by the states, which were far better equipped. For example, health insurance over-sight in California is the responsibility of two agencies: the Department of Insurance, which has over 1,300 employees and is responsible for regulating insurance products sold by over 1,000 carriers, and the Department of Cor-porations, which is responsible for overseeing forty-two full-service health maintenance organizations (HMOs).[8] At any one time, CMS had fewer than fifty full-time employees dedicated to HIPAA oversight and implementa-tion for the entire nation. If California did not want to comply, it would be hard for federal officials to find out; if they did find out, it would be hard to force compliance.

States had the expertise, staff, and systems in place to regulate insurance carriers; CMS did not. CMS was not given the necessary resources and, unlike DOL, could not tap into existing procedures and relationships with the states. Speaking before a Senate committee in 1998, Nancy-Ann Min DeParle, a CMS administrator who later became President Obama's top White House adviser on health care reform, highlighted the agency's staff and resource challenges and also noted that HIPAA tasks had to be done at the same time that the agency was besieged with Medicare and Medicaid changes under the Balanced Budget Act of 1997.[9] She also complained that civil monetary penalties, CMS's main compliance tool, might not be enough to enforce the law and stated that CMS needed "the range of tools utilized by the state insurance agencies" to do so.[10]

In July 1998, CMS had just thirty-nine employees working on HIPAA, seventeen in the central office and twenty-two in four regional offices.[11] Staff members were reassigned from other positions, and most had "no previ-ous experience in private health insurance."[12] In March 2000, CMS said that it had enough staff to fulfill its mission, although the number of staff at that point was down to thirty-one full-time employees and one half-time employee.[13] A review of CMS's progress raised serious questions about the accuracy of that assessment.

In 1998 Congress provided CMS with a supplemental appropriation of $2.2 million for HIPAA oversight and implementation. Most of the money, $1.7 million, was spent on outside contractors, and most of that on actu-arial support. Some of the money ($615,000) was spent conducting a market analysis of what was actually going on in the states. CMS did not build the long-term internal infrastructure necessary for direct oversight, and that lack of infrastructure and experience, combined with the diverse regulatory envi-ronments the states, makes it easy to understand why CMS was in no hurry to find states out of compliance. In practice, federal officials either simply pleaded with states to comply or were content to be left in the dark.

The senior staff of the National Governors Association (NGA), though often critical of CMS, sympathized with its plight. Matt Salvo, NGA's director for health legislation, observed that "CMS did not even have enough resources or staff to do the things that they needed to do before the addition of HIPAA." He added, "They are just now getting around to looking at the states and seeing what they are doing now, four years later. This is clearly an unfunded mandate on CMS."[14] A senior staff member of the National Conference of State Legislatures (NCSL) confirmed that assessment, saying that "the federal government does not have the administrative infrastructure to be able to handle much at all, and it has not in the past."[15]

CMS OVERSIGHT

With the CMS central office unable to take the lead in HIPAA oversight, the job fell to the regional offices. But in one state after another, oversight was not a high priority. The central office did hold a yearly conference with regional office staff and held weekly conference calls to deal with policy issues and identify local problems. Those efforts were largely reactive, and CMS never did push for close examination of state-by-state compliance. According to a GAO report, CMS worried that any aggressive monitoring could "disrupt a market that states had traditionally regulated."[16] CMS also noted that the law requires "substantial"—not "absolute"—compliance.[17] It was legalese in action. Although CMS claimed that it was taking an approach of "collaborative federal-state enforcement of HIPAA-related laws," the GAO provided evidence that federal enforcement efforts were slow, passive, and deferential.[18]

CMS knew early in the game that five states were not following HIPAA rules. Three states—Missouri, California, and Rhode Island—reported to CMS that they were out of compliance with HIPAA rules and that they were unlikely to pass the state legislation necessary to comply. Two additional states, Michigan and Massachusetts, were widely known to be out of compliance. But the list did not end there: a 1998 GAO report concluded that seventeen other states had not enacted laws to "enforce one or more HIPAA provisions."[19] However, CMS took direct enforcement action only when it could no longer avoid doing so, and in this case it managed to avoid taking action quite well. By May 1999, "CMS had yet to comprehensively evaluate the extent to which the other 45 states not known to be out of compliance conformed to HIPAA."[20]

CMS undertook direct enforcement efforts in the three states that voluntarily admitted that they were out of compliance.[21] But the agency did not move against Michigan or Massachusetts, claiming that it had limited resources and was not prepared for the lengthy procedures that would be involved. Regulations required states to be given an official preliminary determination of noncompliance, a forty-five-day period to respond, and additional time for corrective action before federal enforcement began.[22]

Each of the five states known to be noncompliant already had some protections in the small group and individual insurance markets. Some were generally stronger than HIPAA required, but they fell short on certain details. For example, none of the five states required that certificates of creditable coverage be issued. California and Missouri did not guarantee access to insurance in the individual market that was free of pre-existing condition exclusions. The definition of "small business" in Rhode Island, Missouri, and Michigan also was less generous than the federal standard.[23]

Tellingly, many officials at the state level started calling out for more federal involvement. Jay Angoff, the director of the Missouri Department of Insurance, testified before Congress that he thought that Missouri consumers would be better off with federal enforcement since the state legislature seemed unable to agree on a course of action. He noted that under state law, CMS had broader authority to issue regulations than the Missouri Department of Insurance.[24] CMS made some progress working closely with Missouri insurance commission staff, who actually helped train CMS regional office staff to conduct insurance carrier policy reviews. By 1997, Missouri had HIPAA protections through a federal regulatory structure that still relied heavily on state insurance commission staff to guide the federal officials ostensibly in charge.[25] Rhode Island eventually passed appropriate legislation as part of a broader state health care reform package, and CMS, to the state's relief, took no further action.

CMS did the bare minimum to address concerns. By July 1998, CMS had responded to inquiries and complaints in all five states and provided some guidance to carriers in California, Missouri, and Rhode Island. In Missouri, CMS obtained voluntary reporting by nine of the largest carriers in the group and individual markets.[26] By May 1999, CMS developed guidelines and held informational meetings with carriers in Missouri and Rhode Island. The GAO concluded that the CMS was hardly getting aggressive, noting that "enforcement . . . remains largely complaint driven except for policy reviews in Missouri, where carriers voluntarily submit policies for review."[27] Because consumers were largely unaware of these complicated provisions, they were not in a position to complain, leaving CMS blissfully ignorant of major problems.

However, CMS did hire a contractor to conduct onsite examinations in Missouri. Several insurance carriers were notified of potential civil monetary fines, and CMS negotiated with them to pay certain disputed claims. But that was not much more than a token gesture. In March 2000, the GAO reported to Congress that federal enforcement in noncompliant states was "slow." After four years, the GAO concluded that "HCFA continues to be in the early stages of fully identifying where federal enforcement will be required."[28] (HCFA, the Health Care Financing Administration, later became the Centers for Medicare and Medicaid Services.)

CMS administrator DeParle pointed out that by necessity, CMS relied on "information provided voluntarily by states, surveys performed by others, and anecdotal reports."[29] In 1998, the GAO confirmed that "because states were not required to report plans for enforcing most HIPAA standards, HHS has had to rely on information provided voluntarily by the states, surveys performed by others, and anecdotal reports to determine the status of state legislative activity."[30]

The CMS state review in 1999 tracked compliance not only with HIPAA but also with the Mental Health Parity Act, the Newborns' and Mothers' Health Protection Act, and the Women's Health and Cancer Rights Act. States were placed into one of three categories: those that appeared to have acceptable laws; those that had questionable laws; and those that appeared to lack acceptable laws. Twenty-one states fit into the third category.[31] In 2000, the GAO reported that CMS was still moving slowly in enforcing requirements in noncompliant states; unsurprisingly, CMS responded that it was trying to work with the states. In 2004, CMS moved responsibility for HIPAA oversight back to the central office, with the exception of two dedicated full-time regional staff in Kansas City.[32] CMS was figuratively and literally distancing itself further from direct oversight of state insurance reform.

Christie Ferguson, director of Rhode Island Health and Human Services, summarized the situation, noting that "CMS and HHS do not really understand what marketplace regulation is really about and are not investing in the staff to do it." States were concerned about federal preemption, Ferguson said, "but, the reality is that unless they [CMS] come in to some places, HIPAA is not going to be enforced." She added, "I think the danger with HIPAA is that while the intent was clear, the implementation of it has been very weak because it again put new regulatory roles into government, but did not fund them." She noted that CMS officials sent mixed signals "about whether or not they really wanted it done" and that "they could have chosen to implement this in a strong way, but they did not."[33] Although HIPAA theoretically represented an encroachment on state authority by federal authority, in practice the federal government never exercised its authority.

STATE ACTION

Implementation of HIPAA was a complicated undertaking. Responsibility for implementation was split among three federal agencies, fifty states, hundreds of insurers, and thousands of businesses. Similarly but on a grander scale, the Affordable Care Act builds on public and private health care systems that vary significantly by state. With HIPAA, the best predictor of state action was what a state had already accomplished prior to enactment of HIPAA. In other words, the legislation itself did little to expand access to health insurance protections. Federal agencies, particularly CMS, went into implementation blind, with no clear mechanisms for tracing state action and compliance in the small group and individual markets.

Group Market

As discussed, new regulations in the group market require guaranteed issue, guaranteed renewal, and limits on coverage exclusions for preexisting medical conditions. The history of HIPAA has been marked by strong compliance by large employers, mixed compliance in the small group market, and lots of uncertainty. The GAO reported that implementing HIPAA insurance regulations was relatively easy for large group plans because in those plans, many of the protections were already in place.[34] For example, less than half of all group health plans with more than 200 employees had preexisting condition exclusions.[35] Large companies' greatest concern was the administrative burden entailed in the requirement to issue certificates of coverage for former employees and their dependents. It was also reported that there was some success in applying the preexisting condition rule to ERISA plans exempt from state law.[36]

Small group market regulations varied significantly depending on state policy prior to HIPAA. Some states developed new small group market insurance regulations, while the majority complied with minimum statutory changes. Thirteen states, including four of the largest (California, Texas, New York, and Florida), had guaranteed issue and renewability provisions equal to or more protective than HIPAA in the small group market.[37] However, in 1999 the GAO reported that although most states were thought to be in compliance, some had not adopted certificate requirements or a definition of "small group" consistent with HIPAA rules.[38] All but one state and the District of Columbia had small group protection prior to HIPAA. However, many did not have the same definition of "small group": eighteen did not apply protections to groups as large as fifty employees, and thirteen did not count companies with just two employees. Furthermore, only nineteen states gave credit for previous coverage, and no state required automatic issuance of coverage certificates.[39] Overall, thirty-eight states' definition of "preexisting condition" did not match the definition required by federal law.[40]

One early review of HIPAA found that considerable progress had been made by states in enacting conforming legislation but that progress was based on the fact that "states had already enacted significant reforms in the small group and individual insurance market."[41] NAIC also reported progress but noted possible problems with guaranteed issue in several states.[42] The data were just not available, which was a big part of the problem. CMS had no proactive system in place for monitoring state compliance. Accordingly—shock of all shocks—implementation was really successful only in states that already had policies in place that met the new standards.

The GAO reported that 46 percent of insurance agents said that there was increased access to and choice among a wider variety of plans. However, 44 percent of agents agreed that HIPAA did not improve access for small groups and that people in high-risk groups still could not afford coverage.[43] Further, insurance carriers reported an increase in premiums that may or may not have been related to HIPAA.[44] On the other hand, a Kaiser Family Foundation study found that the use of preexisting condition exclusions in small businesses fell in the first two years from 59 to 40 percent and for larger businesses from 62 to 38 percent; the study speculated that the drop was linked in part to HIPAA regulations. At the same time, however, the number of small firms offering insurance declined from 59 to 54 percent. The most common explanation for dropping coverage: increasingly expensive premiums.[45]

Thus, HIPAA's impact in the group market was uncertain. Larger groups had relatively few problems complying with group-to-group portability provisions. The small group market was more complicated. Although most states passed the required legislation, limited data were available to assess insurance carrier or health plan compliance. Outside studies suggested that increased access to health insurance was contingent on state regulation of premium prices.[46] HIPAA was not that strong to begin with, the rule weakened it, and implementation was ultimately left to the discretion of the states.

Individual Market

In the individual insurance market, states could create their own safeguards, implement a "federal fallback" plan, or have the federal government come in and take over the implementation process. Most states simply used their existing individual market insurance programs as an alternative mechanism and achieved compliance with only minor modifications. In total, thirty-eight states chose to implement alternative mechanisms. In all but one of those states, consumer access and protection were "very similar to what existed prior to HIPAA."[47] Twenty-two of the thirty-eight states used high-risk pools that grouped difficult-to-insure people together and subsidized their insurance premiums. Thirteen of the states adopted the federal fallback option, but they had a considerable number of problems and limited success in expanding coverage in the individual market. States had significant autonomy, and there was little evidence of federal oversight.

Access and premium rate guarantees in the thirty-eight states implementing alternative mechanisms were similar to protections in place prior to HIPAA. Moreover, most states had standards that exceeded federal requirements. Six of the states offered alternative mechanisms, five offered guaranteed issue if a person had prior group coverage, two guaranteed access through Blue Cross Blue Shield plans, and twenty-two had high-risk pools.[48] All but one of the twenty-two states that had high-risk pools had them before HIPAA, and only small changes were necessary in those states to meet the goals of the statute.[49] Specifically, thirteen of the states increased lifetime maximum benefits, reduced premiums to 200 percent of the standard health insurance rate, and/or exempted federally eligible people from enrollment caps or other waiting periods.[50] One-half of all risk pool states capped premiums at less than 150 percent of the standard health insurance rate, which is below the federally required cap of 200 percent.[51]

For the thirteen states opting to implement federal fallback provisions in the individual market, the carriers had the option to make all plans available, to offer the two most popular policies in the individual market, or to offer high- and low-cost policies that included some type of subsidization. The GAO reported in February 1998 that costs of individual premiums in states with federal fallback programs were between 140 and 600 percent of the cost of standard premiums.[52]

Premium prices varied drastically because price is still tied to risk and people seeking care in the individual market are generally at higher health risk. Two years after implementation, policy premiums ranged from a low of $149 a month for an HMO in California to $951 a month for a preferred provider plan with a $500 deductible in the District of Columbia.[53] At a congressional hearing, Senator Jim Jeffords (R-Vt.) said that "with rates of this magnitude, I'm not sure you can still call it insurance."[54] It was no surprise that the GAO concluded that "carrier marketing activities and high premium prices may limit consumers' ability to take advantage of this guarantee."[55]

Some insurance carriers in fallback states went to great—and even devious—lengths to discourage HIPAA-eligible individuals from buying insurance. Among other things, they would delay processing applications beyond the sixty-three days allowed for a gap in coverage and falsely report on the range of availability of insurance products. Insurance companies even cut back or eliminated commissions to agents who sold insurance to people who qualified under HIPAA.[56] The NAIC reported to Congress during implementation hearings that eight states were taking action against such treatment of agents. Kansas considered such treatment a "violation of the state's fair practice statute"; South Dakota issued regulations prohibiting differential commissions; and five other states took similar action.[57] A March 1998 memo from CMS to the states outlined the federal response to reduced commissions and application processing delays.[58] Instead of taking the lead, CMS "*strongly encourage[ed]* states to use their authority to take actions against these practices." CMS said that it would "*carefully monitor*" such practices and would take appropriate enforcement action. This qualified federal bureaucratic legalese signaled federal weakness and continued deference to the states.

Nobody knows how many people secured individual policies as a result of HIPAA, but available data suggest that their ranks were relatively small. The GAO reported that the states had not even made a systematic effort to count "HIPAA eligibles." In twenty states with high-risk pools, approximately 63,000 people were enrolled and roughly 6,500, or 10 percent, were HIPAA eligible.[59] It is possible that some—perhaps most—of those people would have been eligible for state programs before HIPAA. In total, only two states enrolled more than 1,000 HIPAA-eligible individuals.[60]

Very few people qualified for protection in the individual market under HIPAA, and even for those that did there was no assurance that the coverage would be affordable. Clearly, there were significant hurdles to eligibility. An eligible person could not have any other source of health insurance, needed to have had eighteen months of prior health coverage with no gaps longer than sixty-three consecutive days (the most recent coverage being with a group health plan or group health insurer), and have exhausted Consolidated Omnibus Budget Reconciliation Act of 1985 (COBRA) benefits.

One of the few implementation studies conducted on HIPAA concluded that the program fell far short of its goals. The study found that "HIPAA's projected impact on individual coverage may have been overestimated, because in all but a handful of states, federally eligible persons have roughly the same access to coverage following HIPAA's enactment as they did prior to it."[61] In 2001, Dean Rosen, who helped draft HIPAA for Senator Nancy Kassebaum (R-Kans.), discounted federal efforts in the individual market, saying that the market was entirely regulated by the states.[62]

Even after HIPAA became a reality, few people understood what it meant. For example, many people mistakenly believed that they would be able keep the same coverage if they changed jobs, that insurance would be available in the individual market to anyone who did not have coverage, and that HIPAA completely eliminated preexisting condition exclusions.[63] Such false expectations combined with weak federal enforcement raised the possibility that federal efforts in the individual market could have done more harm than good. Unrealistic expectations for HIPAA could have slowed any progress toward real reform.

What Does It All Mean?

The federal agency responsible for implementation largely decides the impact that a policy ultimately has on people. The information and expertise gap between the federal government and the states affects the federal government's ability to achieve uniform national goals. With HIPAA, the contrast between DOL's and CMS's approach to implementation demonstrates the importance of meshing new responsibilities with existing institutional procedures and relationships. DOL had clear, understandable responsibilities and was able to tap into existing systems and resources. CMS, in contrast, had new responsibilities, no existing systems, limited resources, and no desire to set up separate regulatory systems in multiple states. The result was weak oversight, varied implementation, and ineffectual policy. The contrast with the implementation of CHIP could not be sharper.

The contrast between the implementation of HIPAA and of CHIP also demonstrates the importance of both reporting requirements and effective mechanisms for holding states accountable. With HIPAA, CMS had a limited understanding of what was going on in individual states and for the most part relied on secondary sources for information. That put the states in the driver's seat. The HIPAA requirements, such as eliminating preexisting condition exclusions in the individual market, could be enforced or ignored at their discretion. With CHIP, reporting requirements were connected to the provision of federal funds; CMS had a clear picture of what was going on, and the states had strong incentives to comply. CMS focused oversight on priority areas, and states retained considerable flexibility. In both cases, federal authority weakened during the implementation process as states adapted rules to particular circumstances.

Studying how policy is implemented is essential to understanding the power relationship between the federal government and the states. Things are not always as they appear in the legislation, statute, or administrative rule. Both carrots and sticks are critical to ensuring strong federal authority and oversight. With CHIP, federal officials had both; with HIPAA, they had neither. CHIP provided substantial funding to the states, but the money would not flow until CMS approved state plans. CMS made site visits and could take action if states did not comply with CHIP rules. State expenditures were scrutinized and sometimes questioned by federal officials, and there was a real threat that funds would be withheld for improper or noncompliant practices. States also had the flexibility to adapt CHIP to the insurance marketplace, including state Medicaid programs. That bounded flexibility made implementation work in practice.

With HIPAA, there were no such boundaries and no financial incentives for state compliance; moreover, federal officials had very little leverage to compel states or insurance companies to act in accordance with the rules. Furthermore, there was little point to federal officials' finding states out of compliance; the federal threat of takeover was neither real nor threatening. CMS did not have the expertise, desire, or capabilities needed to take over state programs, and it did everything possible to avoid taking over. The federal emperor had no clothes, and everyone knew it. Furthermore, states had more authority to compel action from health insurers and health plans than federal regulators did. States could take insurers' licenses away, but federal officials had only empty threats.

The fate of national reform rests on implementation and on the critical responsibilities of state-based health exchanges and the decisions of states to elect to expand Medicaid programs. Exchanges that work to expand coverage with comprehensive benefits will require major coordination between the federal government and the states. Weak national rules with limited oversight will not accomplish coverage goals; they will instead retain the existing state patchwork of coverage. On the other hand, no state flexibility in implementation also would be a disaster. Since states are beginning from very different places and the ACA builds on current programs, a one-size-fits-all approach would be programmatically impossible and politically suicidal. The only way to get all of the states on the same page and achieve coverage goals is to offer state flexibility, contained within federally prescribed corridors. Finding the right balance requires adequate resources for federal and state administrators, established federal program parameters, reporting requirements, and economic incentives tied to meeting policy goals. There should also be a credible threat to withhold significant funds. The threat of federal takeover will not be enough to move states. A true partnership and real money—either given or taken away—will be required to make reform work.

CHAPTER EIGHT

MASSACHUSETTS
LEADS THE WAY

It may come as a surprise to some on the left, but it is the Bush Administration that made the state of Massachusetts' health-care revolution a reality.

Governor Mitt Romney[1]

Today, the suggestion that a Republican administration had anything to do with Massachusetts health care reform would be more shocking to folks on the right than the left. After President Obama used Massachusetts as a model for national reform, Republican and Tea Party activists started to take a much dimmer view of the scene in Massachusetts. Though George W. Bush did not exactly highlight the fact in his memoir, his administration led the way to reform in Massachusetts by pressuring the state to overhaul its health care system in 2005. Further, the administration explicitly approved key components of the plan that would later be incorporated into Obama's signature health care legislation.

The federal government worked closely with Massachusetts to develop plans for the structure and financing of the overhaul. While Massachusetts helped shape national policy, national health care reform will require some modifications in Massachusetts. The details of the Massachusetts reform—including the role of the federal government and the state's struggles with rulemaking and implementation—provide lessons for implementing national reform.

Passed in 2006, the Massachusetts health care reform was a remarkable success. Thanks to so-called "Romney Care," 98 percent of residents had insurance coverage by 2008, and those gains held steady through the economic downturn.[2] The plan provided greater access to health care services, particularly for low-income residents.[3] Fewer people reported going without necessary care, and there was increased use of prescription drugs and preventive health care services.[4] Major progress was also made in reducing racial and ethnic disparities in access to health care services.[5] However, the plan focused largely on access and did not directly address persistently rising health care costs.[6] Reform did pressure the political system to explore cost containment and health care delivery system reforms—steps that will be essential to maintaining near universal coverage.

Massachusetts reform was based on the principle of shared responsibility. It asked individuals, government, and employers to do their share, and it was unique in that it included an individual mandate requiring anyone who could afford health insurance to purchase it. It also created the Massachusetts Health Care Connector, a forerunner of the health care exchanges required in every state by national reform. After hard-fought negotiations, the Massachusetts reforms ended up being bipartisan, passing both the state house of representatives (155-2) and the senate (37-0), in sharp contrast to the Patient Protection and Affordable Care Act (ACA), which in the end passed entirely along partisan lines and was later repealed by the Republican-controlled House of Representatives.

MEDICAID AND FEDERAL WAIVERS

Massachusetts reform built on a long history of innovative expansions of health care coverage. It grew from the MassHealth program, the state's Medicaid program, which was created through a waiver from the federal government.[7] Some background on Medicaid and the state's waiver is essential to understanding the 2006 reforms. Medicaid is a health insurance program for qualified low-income residents that is run by individual states under federal guidelines. The program is a complex intergovernmental morass, but it provides essential services to many, but not all, of the most vulnerable individuals.[8] The largest group of recipients is poor mothers and children; the program also helps many low-income seniors and people with disabilities. Many other groups are covered at state option.

There is an old adage: "If you have seen one Medicaid program . . . you have seen one Medicaid program." A Medicaid recipient in Minnesota may not be eligible for coverage in Mississippi, or the recipient might be eligible for a very different set of benefits. To keep it all straight, states submit detailed eligibility and coverage plans, which are approved by federal officials. On the basis of those plans, states receive partial federal matching funds, on a

MASSACHUSETTS LEADS THE WAY / 101

sliding scale of between 50 and 76 percent, with less affluent states getting a more generous reimbursement. So when a state like Massachusetts (with a 50 percent match) spends a dollar, the federal government provides 50 cents. Volumes are required to understand just one state's Medicaid program.

To complicate things further, states can apply for a Section 1115 waiver, which allows them to throw out most but not all of the Medicaid rules to create something new. Massachusetts constructed its reform around just such a waiver in 1997, when it was authorized to operate a demonstration program for its Medicaid program, the first step toward the creation of the MassHealth program. The waiver allowed the state to simplify enrollment, require recipients to enroll in managed care programs, and add new eligibility categories, expanding Medicaid coverage by 300,000 people. Under the agreement with the federal government, the plan had to be revenue neutral. That was achieved by requiring most Medicaid recipients to be covered by less expensive managed care plans.[9] The MassHealth program would ultimately cover over 1.4 million of the state's 6.4 million population.[10]

The federal funds included in the Section 1115 waiver became contentious, and the conflict helped propel the 2006 reforms. The initial waiver provided significant supplemental payments to two large safety-net hospitals, Boston Medical Center and Cambridge Health Alliance, which provided disproportionate care to low-income populations. Supplemental payments were designed to mitigate the adverse economic effects on these institutions as the waiver shifted more Medicaid recipients to Medicaid managed care plans. The original waiver also created an uncompensated care pool, which collected money from hospitals and insurers and funneled the money back to hospitals to pay for people who could not pay their bills. By collecting money from payers and paying it back to providers through Medicaid or the pool, the state captures federal matching funds without using any state general tax revenue. Similar financial strategies were used by states to maximize federal revenue and minimize the state share. The Bush administration—spurred by a GAO study in 2002—began to take action against such schemes.[11] In Massachusetts, the federal government, concerned about inadequate oversight and accountability for supplemental and uncompensated care pool payments, demanded change, which precipitated reform.

IMPETUS FOR MASSACHUSETTS REFORM

Health care reform in Massachusetts was enacted for many reasons, including the rising number of uninsured individuals, the governor's presidential ambitions, a strong and well-organized consumer advocacy community, legislative leadership, and the active engagement and support of the health care insurers, providers, and hospitals. But a major impetus was a threat from the federal government to stop matching supplemental and uncompensated care pool payments if the state did not overhaul its system, which put the state at risk of losing $385 million dollars in federal funding annually. As part of the renewal process for the waiver on June 30, 2005, the Centers for Medicare and Medicaid Services made it clear that Massachusetts could no longer receive federal matching funds for supplemental payments to hospitals.

Republican Governor Mitt Romney and Democratic Senator Edward Kennedy, who ran against each other in a very bitter U.S. Senate race in 1994, teamed up to negotiate the waiver renewal with the Bush administration. Their goal was to find a way to allow Massachusetts to keep the $385 million. This left-right combination applied political pressure at the highest levels of government. Ultimately, a deal was finalized at a meeting between Kennedy, Romney, and Secretary of Health and Human Services Tommy Thompson on Thompson's last day in office. During negotiations, the secretary's going-away party was under way on the next floor. After the deal was signed, Thompson brought this political "odd couple" to the festivities. They were the hit of the party.[12]

The arrangement outlined a framework for retaining the money by shifting funds to direct coverage of the uninsured. It was all contingent on the state's passage of comprehensive reform, which at the time was still a long shot. The Bush administration's view was that Massachusetts could keep the supplemental funds if, first, it expanded coverage through private health plans without expanding Medicaid and, second, shifted funds away from institutions and instead provided sliding-scale premium support directly to recipients.

The political process shifted to the state. Governor Romney introduced his plan, including health care exchanges and the individual insurance mandate, in April 2005. Attention then focused on the competing plans of Salvador DiMasi, the speaker of the house, and Robert Travaglini, the president of the senate. The Blue Cross Blue Shield of Massachusetts Foundation held a series of events entitled "The Road Map to Coverage." Important forums featuring major policy addresses by the governor, the house speaker, and the senate president were held at the John F. Kennedy Library; the events were attended by the top health care leaders in the state, and they received widespread media coverage. Events included the presentation of commissioned research by the Urban Institute that described the number and characteristics of the uninsured and the cost of various options for covering their health care.[13] The research also concluded that no plan within the current system could get close to universal coverage without an individual mandate,[14] a finding that helped diminish opposition to the mandate, which came mainly from the political left.

State advocacy organizations ratcheted up the political pressure for reform by introducing their own plan. With grassroots support, they collected enough signatures to force a universal health care initiative on the ballot. The driving force behind the campaign was a coalition known as ACT! (Affordable Care Today), led by the advocacy organization Health Care for All.[15] ACT! included labor unions, community health centers, public health advocates, and the Greater Boston Interfaith Organization. The inclusion of faith-based organizations into a coordinated strategy for universal health care broadened and energized the base of support.

The Massachusetts house and senate passed drastically different versions of reform, and the legislation became stalled in a conference committee convened to work out the differences. The house bill was more progressive, aiming for near universal coverage and requiring all but the smallest employers that did not cover their employees to pay a 5 to 7 percent payroll tax. It also included the creation of the exchange—called the "Connector"—and the implementation of the individual mandate found in the governor's bill. The senate bill would have covered far fewer people and included minor contributions from employers.

The state missed its January 15, 2006, deadline for the waiver renewal. Although Massachusetts received an extension, the prospects for reform did not look promising. The house speaker and senate president, both Italian Americans from old Boston neighborhoods who happened to be good friends, stopped talking to each other. In an effort to get things back on track, Senator Kennedy visited the Massachusetts house of representatives and ended up addressing both chambers. Including personal remarks about his family, he spoke of the importance of health insurance to everyone in the commonwealth. Still, there was no progress. On a Sunday that January, a frustrated Governor Romney hand-delivered letters to the homes of the speaker and the senate president urging them to keep working. Senate president Travaglini answered the door in a sweat suit and slippers;[16] speaker DiMasi was not home, so the governor taped the letter to his door. DiMasi and Romney would have a rare closed-door meeting several weeks later. Talks finally revived after the wives of Travaglini and DiMasi invited them to dinner at a restaurant in Boston's North End and urged them to get their acts together.

Establishing the role of business in health care reform proved to be the real obstacle to reform; by comparison, the individual mandate was surprisingly straightforward and noncontroversial. Business leaders, including big players Blue Cross Blue Shield of Massachusetts and Partners Health Care System, helped broker a deal with the help of the Massachusetts Taxpayers Association. The idea was to require businesses having eleven or more full-time employees that did not provide a health insurance plan to pay an annual $295 "fair share" assessment for each uninsured employee, an amount equal to the average amount that employers who provided insurance paid into the state's free-care pool. Blue Cross Blue Shield of Massachusetts and Partners contributed substantially to a media campaign to defend the plan from attack. The plan won critical support from health care advocacy groups, and the business opposition that defeated past attempts at reform started to fade. The legislature embraced the compromise, and the bill was signed on April 12, 2006, at historic Faneuil Hall in a ceremony complete with a colonial fife-and-drum corps.

The deal still had to be approved by the federal government; the waiver, after all, put the feds on the hook for a significant portion of the costs. Kennedy and Romney once again took the lead with senior Bush administration officials, while staff negotiated the details with CMS. Secretary of Health and Human Services Michael Leavitt ultimately approved the waiver despite the fact that the administration was on record as opposing expansion of Medicaid and CHIP to cover people at higher income levels, fearing that doing so could displace private insurance and lead to a government-run health care system. State officials responded to those concerns by invoking the deal originally negotiated with Secretary Thompson.

Success was achieved in part because of the close relationship between Governor Romney and Secretary Leavitt. In fact, when Leavitt was governor of Utah, he hired Romney to run the 2002 Salt Lake City Winter Olympics. Federal officials were also happy that the state would finally reduce supplemental and free-care pool payments. The individual mandate was embraced by Republicans, who had long seen it as an alternative to the type of health care reform proposed by President Clinton in 1994.[17] The Romney administration made the case that Massachusetts reform was founded on conservative principles; in fact, the idea of the exchange came from the conservative Heritage Foundation. Romney characterized the individual mandate as "the ultimate conservative idea, which is that people . . . don't want government to take care of them if they can afford to take care of themselves."[18]

The Massachusetts waiver enabling reform was renewed once again by the Bush administration in 2008 when the state demonstrated that it had in fact reduced supplemental payments and uncompensated care and that money that had been going directly to hospitals was now subsidizing individual insurance. At that time, Secretary Leavitt boasted that "the agreement builds on the Bush Administration's ongoing commitment of helping Massachusetts decrease the number of uninsured individuals while at the same time directing taxpayer dollars to beneficiaries. This helps provide patients with choice and responsibility in obtaining the coverage that best suits their health care needs."[19]

DETAILS

Massachusetts reform expanded Medicaid coverage to children whose family income was up to 300 percent of the federal poverty level ($55,590 for a family of four in 2011). It also created the Commonwealth Care Program, which provided a range of other health insurance options to uninsured adults whose income was up to 300 percent of the poverty level ($32,670 for an individual in 2011). Commonwealth Care subsidies are provided on a sliding scale, with no premiums for families with income below 150 percent of the federal poverty level (FPL) and sliding-scale premiums for people with income between 150 and 300 percent of the poverty level. Federal subsidies under the ACA will cover the full premium for incomes of up to 133 percent of the FPL ($29,726 for a family of four in 2011), with somewhat less generous sliding-scale support for incomes of up to 400 percent of the FPL ($89,400 for a family of four in 2011). However, while Massachusetts subsidies go directly to pay for Commonwealth Care plan premiums, national subsidies will take the shape of tax credits.[20]

The state's Commonwealth Health Insurance Connector Authority (the Connector) was designed to take over some of the key tasks of health care reform, including running the Commonwealth Care and Commonwealth Choice programs. Commonwealth Care provides subsidies to qualified people and offers them a choice of health plans. Here the Connector is an active purchaser of services, negotiating premiums primarily with Medicaid managed care providers. It has been successful in keeping costs below private market prices. Commonwealth Care enrolls over 300,000 people in five plans.

The other arm of the Connector, Commonwealth Choice, is more like the exchange envisioned by the ACA. The idea is to provide an online portal, similar to trip-booking sites like Travelocity.com, to allow consumers to compare health plans on cost and quality before purchase. Massachusetts merged the individual and small group insurance markets, making Commonwealth Choice available to uninsured individuals and small businesses with fifty or fewer employees. However, it has been more successful in covering uninsured individuals than in covering many small businesses. Commonwealth Choice also makes a limited benefit plan available to young adults. Plans are offered in gold, silver, and bronze options. Benefits in each category are similar; the differences lie in the premiums and copayments. The gold plan has a higher premium but covers a greater percentage of medical costs and has lower out-of-pocket costs. The bronze plan has lower monthly premiums but higher out-of-pocket costs. The silver plan is between the two on both dimensions. Plans were named after Olympic medals in part because of Governor Romney's work on the 2002 Winter Olympics in Salt Lake City. The ACA has since added a fourth option, the platinum plan, that has even lower premiums.

The individual mandate to buy insurance applies only to people who can afford it, as defined by the state's affordability schedule. The penalty for being uninsured is half the price of the lowest-cost plan in a particular area. For middle- and higher-income taxpayers over the age 26, the Connector set the amount at $1,116 for someone who went without insurance for all of 2010.[21] Penalties are lower for adults below 26 and for lower-income people. The penalty ended up applying to less than 3 percent of the population, and only 1 percent of taxpayers were actually required to pay the penalty for 2008.[22] The penalty can be waived based on an individual's or family's financial situation. The required benefits are fairly comprehensive, but they are still on par with benefits generally available through employer-based coverage in the state. In contrast, the federal penalty for not having insurance in 2016 will be the greater of $695 or 2.5 percent of income, capped at $2,085; that amount will be adjusted for inflation over time.

In the Massachusetts plan, employers not providing insurance are required to pay a "fair share assessment" of $295 per uninsured employee per year. The fee turned out to be a bargain for such employers, and it ultimately raised less than $20 million in state revenue, which in health care dollars is not much. Because the individual mandate led to many of the previously uninsured signing up for coverage at work, employers who were already providing health insurance ended up making a far greater contribution than their competitors who did not provide insurance. Employers ended up paying a substantial share of the premium for additional employees, at an aggregate cost of well over $750 million.[23]

One of the worries about reform was that employers would simply drop coverage, pay the small fee, and move their employees into the Connector, a shift that would significantly increase the number of people eligible for subsidies and greatly boost the cost of the program. Similar concerns have been expressed for national reform. But that did not happen in Massachusetts. In fact, the state saw a slight increase in the number of employers offering health insurance at a time when employer coverage nationwide actually dropped.[24]

But the fear remains. Business people that I speak to around the country often tell me that their competitors would rather pay the fee than provide health insurance. But there are sound reasons why that never happened in Massachusetts. Employers offer insurance to attract and retain good employees. The individual coverage mandate makes health insurance a value-added offering for employers.

REGULATION AND IMPLEMENTATION

As with CHIP and HIPAA, many of the key implementation issues in Massachusetts were left to the rulemaking process. The Connector Board—which consisted of ten members, selected by the governor and the attorney general, representing labor, business, and consumers and included top government officials—was responsible for developing the Massachusetts health care reform rules. Major responsibilities included the following:

—developing and running the Commonwealth Care Insurance Program

—developing and running the Commonwealth Choice Program

—providing a "seal of approval" for health plans offered through the Connector

—establishing young adult plans for people between 19 and 26 years of age

—defining the minimum health insurance coverage (minimum creditable coverage) required to meet the mandate

—creating an affordability standard

—developing rules for implementing the individual mandate

—supporting public outreach and awareness

—creating a business strategy to be financially self-sustaining

—becoming a health care broker and purchasing agent.

The legislation did not define several essential elements, including what was "affordable" for the purpose of the individual mandate or even what constitutes "insurance." Such fundamental questions were left to the Connector Board for the same reasons that, in a democracy, legislation often is ambiguous. First, those are difficult technical questions. Second, filling in the details might have unraveled the delicate political coalition necessary for passage. For example, no politician wants to tell chiropractors, or any other provider group, that their services will not be covered. With ambiguous legislation, the politician can hide behind the board. Here a legislator could tell providers in her city, "I understand how valuable your services are, and I certainly would have included them if I could have."

Because they determine how resources are allocated—essentially who wins and who loses—such decisions take on a deeply political dimension.

All Connector meetings were open to the public. While that led to some loud arguments and tense negotiations, public input added credibility to the solutions. Having business, labor, and consumer organizations come to a consensus on challenging questions of affordability and benefits was as critical as the actual decision made. Under the ACA, the subsidies have already been defined, but the essential benefits package is still to be determined. Interest groups and the public may never have the input—or the sense of ownership—that helped make Massachusetts reform a reality.

AFFORDABILITY

One of the most critical decisions that the Connector Board made concerned the precise definition of "affordable insurance," which determines whom the individual mandate applies to and who will pay a penalty for remaining uninsured. There are trade-offs in setting this standard. Exempting many people from the mandate would lead to lower coverage levels, but requiring insurance for people who cannot afford it is unfair and politically unpopular. Consumer groups wanted to exempt far more people from the mandate than the business community did. In the end, the Connector Board found the middle ground by increasing subsidy levels to make coverage more affordable at lower income levels and including individual exemptions to account for unique circumstances across the income spectrum. As part of that process, the Connector Board increased the family income level required to receive a full premium subsidy from 100 to 150 percent of the FPL. Since most of the people on Commonwealth Care are receiving full subsidies, that increased enrollment and coverage at the lower end of the income scale.

The Connector Board used analysis and data from consumer groups, economists, and policy analysts to make what was ultimately a political decision. An economist on the board ran simulation models estimating what people at certain income levels were already spending on health care.[25] The Greater Boston Interfaith Organization collected information from church focus groups examining people's bills to determine whether they could afford to pay for health insurance.[26] The board also used information about affordability standards for other social welfare benefits, like CHIP. That research and analysis was used in the process of bargaining and negotiating among stakeholders, which ultimately led to a consensus. Consumer groups did not get all that they wanted, and they could have put pressure on the Connector Board by threatening to publicly denounce the mandate as draconian. The business community could have done the same thing, characterizing the mandate as too weak to achieve coverage goals. But because all parties

Table 8-1. *Premium Affordability for an Individual, by Income Range, 2010*

Income (dollars)	Affordable monthly premium	Percent of family income at the midpoint[a]
0–16,248	$0	0 percent
16,248–21,660	$39	2.5 percent
21,661–27,084	$77	3.8 percent
27,085–32,496	$116	4.7 percent
32,497–39,000	$175	5.9 percent
39,001–44,200	$235	6.7 percent
44,201–54,600	$354	8.6 percent
54,600 +	Always affordable	

Source: Commonwealth Health Insurance Connector Authority.

a. This is the percent of income (measured at the midpoint of the range of numbers in the first column) that the monthly premium represents.

wanted reform to succeed, the consumer groups and the business community compromised and kept working toward consensus. The process itself aided in ensuring the legitimacy of the standard, and it was essential to retain stakeholder support and limit opposition to the mandate.

The decision required people to spend a larger portion of their income on health insurance as their income increased. Premiums are free for people at or below 150 percent of FPL ($33,525 for a family of four in 2011), but people making over 500 percent of FPL ($111,750 for a family of four in 2011) pay the full amount. The board created subsidy levels for Commonwealth Care for people with incomes of up to 300 percent of FPL, as shown in table 8-1.

BENEFITS

Before Massachusetts could mandate insurance, it had to define the very term. What type of insurance would satisfy the requirements of the mandate? Would a high-deductible, catastrophic coverage–only plan suffice? What about a bare-bones plan that ended after, say, $2,000 worth of coverage? Such limited-benefit plans are widespread at major fast food chains and discount stores. Further, what benefits need to be included for a person to be considered "covered" for the purposes of the mandate? For example, would prescription drug coverage be required? Some employer-provided plans in Massachusetts did not already include that kind of coverage. So, if drug coverage was required, would those people be considered uninsured and subject to the penalty? As it turned out, the answer to the last question was yes. Some people who thought that they had health insurance were actually uninsured in the eyes of the state.

In Massachusetts, the Connector Board decided that a comprehensive set of benefits should be required to meet the standards of minimum creditable coverage (MCC). They include the following:

—hospital, physician, and other provider services, including diagnostics
—mental health parity
—prescription drug coverage
—annual out-of-pocket cap of $5,000 for an individual and $10,000 for a family
—deductibles cannot exceed $2,000 per individual and $4,000 per family unless combined with a medical savings account
—coverage of preventive care physician visits must be provided prior to any deductible
—no limits on coverage per year or per sickness.

So, if a person in Massachusetts has insurance that covers everything but, say, preventive care physician visits prior to the deductibles, he is considered uninsured for the purposes of the mandate and is subject to the tax penalty.

The Connector Board had to make some important trade-offs to establish the required benefits package. On one hand, mandating comprehensive benefits requires people to buy something very expensive and could force them to choose between paying for comprehensive coverage or essentials such as food and rent or, alternatively, going without insurance and paying the penalty. If plans are too costly, the financial sustainability of the program could be at risk. On the other hand, allowing slimmed-down benefits or very high-deductible catastrophic plans may simply replace uninsured people with underinsured people. In that case, it is easy to imagine a person's frustration at diligently paying monthly premiums and then having to pay significant additional fees every time he or she uses services or finding out that the services needed are not covered. That services are not covered does not mean that they are not necessary.

One of the promises of near-universal coverage is that individuals will get the care that they need without falling deep into debt. Another is that hospitals and providers will no longer be saddled with unpaid bills. Those promises remained in doubt during the rulemaking process. In the end, requiring near-comprehensive coverage worked in part because it was in keeping with the insurance that most people already had.

For all of its successes, Massachusetts reform did not rein in high insurance costs. The long-term future of the plan rests on bringing these costs under control. Instead of reducing costs by cutting benefits, the state is considering ways to increase the efficiency of the health care delivery system. In 2009, the Massachusetts Special Commission on the Health Care Payment System (Special Commission) recommended restructuring the payment system to promote efficiency while reducing costs and improving quality.[27] The study, conducted with broad interest group consensus, concluded that the current fee-for-service payment system rewards volume instead of positive outcomes and efficiency. In other words, if hospitals are paid on the basis of the number of operations, MRIs, and other procedures that they perform, doctors are more likely to recommend aggressive, expensive treatments when a more conservative approach might be better for the patient. This system also discourages preventative care that might help keep a person from getting sick in the first place.

The Special Commission called for Massachusetts to address these problems by transitioning toward alternative payment models, such as global or bundled payments. Instead of paying piecemeal for each service or procedure, lump payments might be made to an accountable care organization (ACO) composed of physicians and other providers. It is argued that this model may encourage health organizations to scrimp on services, but if organizations are held to measurable quality standards, there is a real possibility that care could be improved while costs decrease. The idea is to align the incentives of providers, payers, and patients to keep people healthy. The current situation certainly leaves considerable room for improvement. Other nations spend a lot less than the United States but enjoy far better health outcomes.[28] Even though hospitals, physician groups, consumer advocates, and current Massachusetts governor Deval Patrick have all signed off on this plan, it will be far more difficult to achieve than reform because any savings from cost reductions will curtail someone's revenue.

COMPARISONS WITH THE NATION

While health care reform in Massachusetts was still a major undertaking, the state had a number of advantages that many other states do not enjoy. The number of uninsured people that Massachusetts began with was low (10 percent) compared with the national average (16 percent). It had a relatively high percentage of people covered by employer-provided insurance.[29] It had resources from the uncompensated care pool and supplemental payments that could be shifted to help pay for expansion of coverage. The state had a history of reform, and the major interest groups and consumer advocacy groups already had working relationships.[30] Massachusetts already had enacted progressive insurance market regulations, including modified community ratings in the individual insurance market, which meant that insurance premiums could vary only by age and region. The state also requires health insurance coverage to be comprehensive, and it has relatively fewer very high-deductible plans than other states. The state health insurance industry is dominated by nonprofit organizations recognized nationally for their quality.[31] Reform had broad bipartisan support that assuaged business opposition. Finally, at the time of passage, the state was enjoying strong economic growth, low unemployment, and a budget surplus.

Enrollment of the uninsured, one of the biggest hurdles in the national reform process, happened relatively quickly in Massachusetts. The state already had lists of people enrolled in the free-care program that could be transferred to Commonwealth Care. The state ran a major advertising campaign on multiple levels; for example, the Red Sox were used to spread the word about the requirement to obtain insurance. At the grassroots level, the state provided small dollar grants to not-for-profit agencies to go in the neighborhoods to talk peer to peer about the mandate and the range of subsidized insurance that was available. The state facilitated enrollment through a universal intake system known as the "virtual gateway" that screens for eligibility for MassHealth, Commonwealth Care, and Safety Net Care (the residual free-care pool) in addition to other social programs including WIC (Women, Infants, and Children), SNAP (the Supplemental Nutrition Assistance Program, formerly the Food Stamp Program), and a host of other services. The gateway can be accessed online, at government offices, and through third parties at hospitals and community health centers. In 2009, over 4,000 people in 248 hospitals assisted individuals and families with applications for health assistance programs.[32]

Implementing national reform in states without such advantages will be far more challenging. For example, Texas begins with an uninsured population of more than 25 percent and a far wider range of existing health plans, many with benefits that fall far short of what the ACA is likely to require. Implementation will be further complicated by strong political opposition from Texas politicians and interest groups. Many states also have far weaker safety nets in that their Medicaid and CHIP programs leave the majority of their low-income residents uninsured. Many states also have more limited insurance regulations and will have a much greater distance to travel to comply with new federal rules regarding preexisting conditions and rate regulations.

Furthermore, the Obama administration is likely to take a fairly comprehensive view of the term "essential benefits." As justified as this may be for the overall health of the nation, it will be difficult to realize in practice. While the ACA has a grandfather clause that exempts insurance that employers are currently providing, plans will have to be upgraded to meet the new standards, and that requirement could lead to economic challenges and renewed political opposition. Already there is both a wide range of political support and outright opposition to "Obamacare." More than twenty states joined in the lawsuit against the individual mandate, which, if it had been successful, would have effectively killed large sections of the ACA. Florida has refused to accept grant money to begin constructing state health care exchanges. Louisiana, along with a majority of states, declared that it will not establish health care exchanges and will instead leave the job to federal officials. These states are unlikely to do the outreach necessary to cover hard-to-reach populations. All these factors will make an already challenging implementation process more difficult.

LESSONS FOR NATIONAL REFORM

National reform builds on existing health care systems, which vary dramatically among states. Implementing national reforms state by state on this uneven base will be a monumental challenge. A number of lessons can be drawn from the Massachusetts experience. First, it takes more than a law alone to make an individual mandate work; the standard for affordability needs to be reasonable and legitimate too. Massachusetts achieved that through a process of bargaining and negotiating among stakeholders, including consumer advocates. Second, significant marketing and outreach will be necessary to inform the public about the mandate, the available coverage options, and the range of subsidies. Mass advertising is important, but peer-to-peer efforts that are culturally and linguistically appropriate are essential. They can be conducted with small grants to existing organizations. Since the cost for many new low-income enrollees will be paid for predominantly with federal money, this cost may be easier for states to justify. Third, states need an enrollment process that is open and accessible, with multiple options for people to get assistance with the transition to subsidized coverage. Assistance should be available at the point where people seek care, including hospitals and health centers as well as government offices and community centers. Reductions in employer coverage may not be as big a concern as some anticipate, but states and the federal government should monitor efforts to shift lower-income workers from employer-provided insurance to publicly subsidized coverage.

Establishing and running health insurance exchanges may prove to be the greatest challenge for national reform. There's some reason for optimism, however; the success of Commonwealth Care shows that exchanges can successfully negotiate premiums with insurers and provide greater value to enrollees and the government. But the struggles of Commonwealth Choice indicate that attracting small business to an exchange requires providing lower, more stable premiums. Federal regulations and oversight will need to provide states with the flexibility to adapt exchanges to their existing health care system while moving toward universal comprehensive coverage. Most states do not have the insurance regulations that Massachusetts developed over the years. While states have until 2014 to bring health exchanges online, that will not be enough time for some to institute the insurance regulations necessary to set up a fully functioning exchange.

Another lesson is the importance of public and interest group engagement in the process of establishing health care exchanges and affordability and coverage levels. This is essential both to ensure the legitimacy of the standards and to create broad-based support for the program. It is also critical that health care exchanges demonstrate value to individuals and small businesses. Massachusetts showed a clear benefit to subsidized enrollees in the Commonwealth Care program and to individuals enrolling in Commonwealth Choice. Products were more affordable, and benefits were comprehensive. No such value was demonstrated for small businesses in Commonwealth Choice, and the result can be seen in their meager enrollment.

Massachusetts reform served as a model for the central elements of the ACA, but it is hardly a blueprint for certain success. For one thing, the Massachusetts experiment would not have been possible without the support and financing of the federal government. Even after reform, the state will have to make some adjustments to comply with the ACA. Massachusetts made many mid-course corrections and changes, an experience that will be repeated by every other state during national reform. Adjustments will have to made to federal policy and then again in how to apply policy to particular states. Understanding these intergovernmental dynamics will become even more important to understanding and influencing state and national reform.

CHAPTER NINE

FEDERALISM AND THE AFFORDABLE CARE ACT

Beginning with President Franklin D. Roosevelt's New Deal in the 1930s, Americans began to look to the federal government to remedy some of the country's most pressing social, economic, and environmental ills. The Social Security Act of 1935 created federal pensions, unemployment insurance, and welfare assistance programs. In the 1960s, President Lyndon B. Johnson's War on Poverty and other Great Society–era programs significantly expanded the role and reach of the federal government. Social Security was broadened, welfare assistance expanded, and Medicare and Medicaid were created. Strong environmental standards and regulations were passed, including the Clean Air Act and the Clean Water Act. Congress and the president enacted legislation governing the safety of food and drugs, the minimum wage, workplace conditions, and civil rights. However, all attempts to enact universal health care coverage were thwarted.[1]

Beginning in the 1980s, Ronald Reagan put the brakes on this progressive social welfare agenda. The "liberal" label became an insult, with severe ballot-box consequences for politicians. Not recognizing the magnitude of this seismic political shift, liberals clung to the belief that the federal government was the place to germinate progressive policy change. Democrats played defense, placing hopes in the next election and the emergence of a national political savior in the mold of FDR or LBJ. This strategy protected vital elements of the social safety net, including Social Security, Medicare, and Medicaid, but progressive social welfare policy at the national level was moribund.

The election and governance of President Bill Clinton demonstrated how conservative principles still dominated the American political landscape in contemporary times. Clinton's legislative agenda was actually to the right of that of President Richard Nixon, a Republican who two decades earlier had

115

advocated for the Family Assistance Program, which would have guaranteed a minimum income for all American families. Nixon instituted national wage and price controls on industry and enacted progressive environmental protection legislation. He also advocated for universal health care with a strong employer mandate to provide health insurance.[2]

President Clinton, similar to his predecessor President George H. W. Bush, wanted to be the education president and pushed for volunteerism (Bush had his "Thousand Points of Light" campaign and Clinton had Americorps). Clinton advocated for free trade agreements and passed a welfare reform program that held recipients more accountable by including work requirements and time limits on receipt of benefits. While Ronald Reagan had said that "government isn't the solution, it is the problem," Bill Clinton announced that "the era of big government is over." One major exception was Clinton's health care proposal, which suffered a stunning defeat. Reducing poverty and advocating for national policies to expand opportunity to the most vulnerable remain a losing political issue in the United States. President Obama seeks to be the great reconciler-in-chief, bringing together the political left and right to address the nation's economic crisis. And while the economic stimulus package included significant funding for infrastructure and enhanced funding for the states, the government's bailout of the banks and support of Wall Street sustained to a large degree President George W. Bush's policies. Despite his largely moderate record and agenda, President Obama is decried on the right as a "socialist." Tea Party backers are convinced of it, progressives wish it were at least a little bit true, and Europeans and others with a broader view of the political spectrum find it all a bit comical.

As was Clinton's, the Obama administration's notable progressive social policy initiative was national health care reform. I was a member of the Clinton health care task force—and admittedly part of the problem. The task force presented a fully delineated plan to Congress, leaving interest groups and some key Congressional leaders feeling alienated from the process.[34] In the end, the only people who "owned" the Clinton plan were the Clintons.

But this time, the outcome was different. The Obama administration learned from the defeat of the Clinton plan. First, Obama gave ownership of the process and details to Congress. When Congress creates detailed legislation, it engages interest groups more directly in the process. Although that risks discontinuity, multiplicity of purpose, complexity, and inefficiency, it increases the chance of passage. Second, the Obama administration negotiated directly with interest groups such as the insurance industry and the pharmaceutical industry—groups that help defeat the Clinton plan. Unquestionably, there is a price to pay for engaging the regulated community in the process of reform, but not doing so risks defeat and holds the intended beneficiaries hostage. The Massachusetts reform actively engaged the insurance and hospital industries, the American Medical Association (AMA), and others in a process of compromise and broad stakeholder negotiation.

American politics is no place for the policy purist. The current round of national health care reform is an example of a progressive policy in a conservative era. The question is whether flawed legislation is better than no legislation at all, and the balance is determined by how much has to be sacrificed. While advocates of a single-payer health care system, on the left, and proponents of a voucher system, on the right, may decry such incremental reform, the alternative in the short and medium run is no reform at all.

Obama's plan was subject to the same "socialized medicine" criticism as the Clinton plan, but the claims had less effect because most stakeholders were on board, the structure of reform built on the existing health care system, and a similar plan was already in place in Massachusetts. The ACA, like the Massachusetts plan, will not radically alter the way that most people receive health insurance, as the Clinton plan would have done. Fear of the unknown always trumps the hope that something new will be better, especially when the issue is as personal as health care. Opponents of the Clinton plan could paint a picture of a health care "boogieman" in part because its foundational concept, "managed competition," was new and supporters could not identify an existing success. In contrast, supporters of the ACA could point to Massachusetts, and insurers and other powerful interests could see that this type of reform was not a threat.

CHIP, HIPAA, and the Massachusetts health care reform are all examples of progressive policy germinated in the states and adopted nationally. Other examples include minimum auto fuel efficiency standards, inclusion of nutritional information on fast food chain menus, and regulation of gifts to physicians by the pharmaceutical industry. Fuel efficiency standards were passed nationally after unilateral action by California. Fast food menu labeling and pharmaceutical company gift restrictions were included in the ACA with diminished opposition from food industry groups because a number of places—including California, Maine, Massachusetts, New Jersey, Oregon, New York City, and Philadelphia—already had enacted such requirements and many other states and localities were moving in that direction.[4] Although industry initially fought the laws, once they took root at the state level industry opted to try to influence national policy and forgo rigorous opposition. While generally opposed to regulation, business usually finds consistent, stable national regulation preferable to a range of different state and local standards.

Laws passed at the state level can provide political cover for national action and mitigate cries of "socialism" and "big government takeover." With CHIP, state action was exaggerated to make the point that the federal government was only pursuing a path that the states had already taken. With HIPAA, the idea that states were doing as much or more than what was being considered at the federal level solidified conservative support for action. The ACA could point to the Massachusetts bipartisan effort to temper cries of "socialism." While opponents of reform still made that claim, the argument had less validity and less public appeal.

STATES AS LABORATORIES

As Justice Louis D. Brandeis said, courageous states can serve as "laboratories of democracy" without putting the entire nation at risk. In the current political climate, understanding and consciously applying an intergovernmental strategy may be the best and perhaps the only way to achieve social policy change. With the federal government divided along partisan lines and the current focus on fiscal policy, debt reduction, and mounting deficits, national social policy innovation is unlikely. Advocates of progressive public policy would be wise to stop waiting for a national savior and focus on a more complex intergovernmental strategy. Rather than FDR or LBJ, the role model here is the late Massachusetts senator Edward Kennedy. In the 1960s and 1970s Senator Kennedy was at the forefront in advocating for the most liberal policies, including a single-payer health care system. In the 1980s and 1990s, his goals remained the same, but Kennedy either consciously adopted an incremental strategy or one evolved gradually as he pushed, case by case, for whatever progress was politically possible at the time. Kennedy worked in a bipartisan manner with Senator Orrin Hatch (R-Utah) to pass CHIP, with Senator Nancy Kassebaum (R-Kans.) to pass HIPAA, and with Governor Mitt Romney (R-Mass.) and Bush administration secretaries of health and human services Tommy Thompson and Mike Leavitt to smooth the way for the Massachusetts reforms. In each case, state action was leveraged to nationalize policy. Issues of federalism were used to broaden the political coalition and neutralize arguments about "big government."

However, unilateral state actions may vary greatly and not necessarily comport with national goals. Even the most progressive states will have difficulty sustaining social welfare policy if it is significantly out of step with that of their neighbors. States are required to balance their budgets, and therefore higher taxes for redistributive policies may place them at a competitive disadvantage with their neighbors. One strategy is to germinate social policy change by leveraging federal money for state experiments that, when successful, can serve as national models. This can and is being done through waivers that enable innovation in Medicaid, welfare cash assistance programs, and the creative use of block grant money to address homelessness, substance abuse, teen pregnancy, job training, and community development. Foundations can also effectively target resources to support state experiments as well as to identify and disseminate best practices. CHIP demonstrates that even a small success with state dollars can yield substantial national progress.

When the front door is locked, it is best to try another opening. This strategy is not new. In the ongoing battle over abortion rights, pro-life supporters are using an integrated state and national strategy to weaken the national protection of a woman's right to choose under *Roe* v. *Wade*. They are pushing for legislation at the state level to require a waiting period, parental notification for minors, and other barriers with the explicit long-term goal of changing national policy. In September 2011, a federal court upheld a Kansas law prohibiting abortion services from being offered as part of general health insurance coverage except if the mother's life is in danger.[5] Women will be required to purchase separate coverage just for this service, effectively diminishing access. In October 2011 anti-abortion groups announced plans to introduce legislation in all fifty states requiring a mother to listen to the fetal heartbeat before receiving an abortion.[6] Regardless of where one stands on these issues, understanding this intergovernmental dynamic is essential to understanding the policy process and how it is formed and influenced.

Federalism across the Policy Process

Contemporary social policy is created by the interaction of the federal and state governments throughout the policymaking process, and understanding their interaction is essential to knowing how policy and programs impact people. CHIP, HIPAA, and the Massachusetts reform were all created, shaped, and reshaped through this intergovernmental dance as legislation was developed, rules were written, and programs were implemented and revised. These cases provide insight into how intergovernmental relations might be structured to achieve policy goals. How federalism—the relationship between the federal government and the states with respect to their powers and authority—plays out is influenced by a number of factors.

Federal reporting requirements, incentives, and sanctions strengthen the federal government; their absence strengthens the states and the regulated community. In the very act of implementing a law, states gain the power to shape how a program or policy actually works. Federal control is enhanced if responsibility for a policy is given to a federal agency that has the expertise, routines, and resources needed to write the regulations and hold states accountable during implementation. That was the case with CHIP; the states had real flexibility, but it was circumscribed by federal rules. The combination yielded national accountability with leeway for state innovation, resulting in the coverage of millions of uninsured children.

Conversely, if the states have the expertise, routines, and resources, they will be in a strong position to influence federal legislation and regulations. That was the case with HIPAA. Here the federal government moved into an area reserved for the states, but during the rulemaking and implementation process federal officials abdicated responsibility to the states. Federal officials did not have the economic incentives, technical expertise, or ability to compel state action. The threat of a federal takeover was never a real threat. Ultimately, HIPAA neither delivered on its promise of health care portability nor eliminated preexisting condition exclusions.

The intergovernmental two-step played out differently in Massachusetts. There, the federal government insisted on reform and the state took the initiative and then leveraged federal funds to significantly expand access. In the process, they created a model for national reform, which in turn will require changes by the states, including Massachusetts.

A state policy can be leveraged and its impact exponentially magnified by nationalization of the policy. State expansion of insurance coverage through CHIP, along with federal money and guidance, ultimately extended coverage to millions of uninsured children throughout the nation; that expansion built on nascent state programs that had expanded access to health insurance to just a small fraction of uninsured children. Massachusetts health care reform extended coverage to 400,000 previously uninsured people. The ACA, fully implemented, would cover over 30 million uninsured Americans. One note of caution: HIPAA illustrates that nationalization does not necessarily lead to great uniformity across states or significantly enhanced consumer protections. Elements of national reform, such as health care exchanges, could suffer the same fate.

The location of a program within the federal government matters. The Centers for Medicare and Medicaid Services (CMS), which was committed to making CHIP work and to holding states accountable, drew on institutional routines created by the Medicaid program. States resented being treated like an interest group, especially during the formal rulemaking. They were frustrated with the lack of federal appreciation of the magnitude of work resulting from sometimes insignificant policy changes. CMS got away with it because states supported the program and wanted the enhanced financing.

That may not be the case with the ACA. The contrast between the CMS's oversight of CHIP and the Department of Labor's oversight of HIPAA drives home the importance of institutional routines, administrative resources, and historical capacity. The Department of Labor had a far easier time because its responsibilities coincided nicely with its core mission, existing routines, and relationships with employers. It knew how to do what it was asked to do because it was already doing similar things. Insight into intergovernmental relations throughout the policy process is essential to understanding contemporary health and social welfare policy.

IMPLEMENTING THE AFFORDABLE CARE ACT

Proponents of the ACA should try to implement as much of the legislation as soon as possible, ensure that eligible individuals have access to its benefits, and create a constituency for the changes. The goal should be to put as many stakes in the ground as soon as possible in order to make repeal difficult. Here, the Obama administration has had some early success. The most popular provision was to allow young adults up to the age of 26 to stay on their parents' health insurance plans. Remember Jack's question in chapter 1 about coverage for his daughter Meghan? This provision resulted in the enrollment of close to 1 million people and significantly reduced the number of uninsured individuals between 18 and 26 years of age.[7] It enjoys strong middle- and upper-class support, and it is doubtful that it will ever be repealed, even if the Tea Party dominates all branches of government. Other early provisions include the elimination of preexisting condition exclusions for children, a down payment on filling in a gap in Medicare prescription drug coverage known as the donut hole, and the provision of a range of preventive health care services without requiring copayments. Further, the ACA provides significant tax subsidies to hold small businesses over until exchanges can be brought online.

Opponents want to stall implementation to bolster the claim of inefficient government. They want to prevent the argument from shifting from whether the ACA should be implemented to how it should be implemented. They do not want the states to engage in implementation because doing so will give reform roots and reduce the chances of repeal. Despite the fact that the ACA was not a major campaign issue for President Obama or his challenger, Mitt Romney, the results dealt a major blow to opponents of health reform. With a Democrat-controlled Senate and the president's reelection, short-term repeal is off the table and defunding is more difficult. Just as important, the Obama administration has four more years to write the rules and work with states on implementation. One could imagine far different rules under Romney, whose agenda was to begin with rolling back the ACA "on day one." This said, implementation is still a monumental challenge.

The Supreme Court ruling upholding the individual mandate and the reelection of President Obama kept national health care reform on track. States waited on the sidelines until after the election to make critical decisions about their engagement in implementation. Unlike CHIP, HIPAA, and the Massachusetts health care reform, the ACA was passed along partisan lines. Modifications, particularly if they require increased federal authority or resources, will be blocked by a Republican-controlled House of Representatives, which voted several times in 2012 to repeal the bill. More important, thirty state governors are Republican and twenty-seven states were part of the lawsuit against the individual mandate. Since politics continues into the rulemaking and implementation process, continued opposition, particularly in the states, will be a major hurdle.

The individual mandate is essential to making reform work. Without a mandate, it will be difficult to require insurance companies to cover all who apply and not to drop people from coverage. The Massachusetts reform demonstrated that the individual mandate, along with outreach, helped drive many of the uninsured to Medicaid, the state's health care exchange, employer-sponsored insurance, or the individual private market.[8] As an Urban Institute report noted, universal coverage, or anything close, cannot be achieved without an individual mandate.[9] In Massachusetts, many of the uninsured were previously eligible for Medicaid but signed up only after the mandate. The individual mandate will also capture many of the "young invincibles"—younger adults, primarily male, who can arguably afford insurance but choose not to buy it. But a mandate is reasonable only if subsidies or cost controls make health insurance affordable. It is ludicrous to demand that people pay for something that they cannot afford. Subsidies are provided through Medicaid and health care exchanges, which will be directly shaped by intergovernmental relations.

The Massachusetts experience demonstrates that the mandate and subsidies alone will not be enough to reach coverage targets. The ACA will require a sophisticated multipronged media strategy to let the public know that health insurance is required, where it can be acquired, and what subsidies are available. A 2012 survey by Lake Research Partners found that 78 percent of uninsured people likely to qualify for subsidies in the exchange had no idea that support was going to be available.[10] Another survey found that 83 percent of people who will be eligible for the Medicaid program were unaware of their eligibility for Medicaid.[11] To inform the public, statewide information campaigns will need to be coupled with grassroots and culturally appropriate peer-to-peer education efforts to get close to universal coverage targets.

Further, the enrollment process needs to be easy; there should be multiple places where people can sign up for coverage, including hospitals, community health centers, and websites. While a national campaign might be helpful, most outreach needs to be done at the state level. With the wide variation in states' support and capacity, the best strategy may be to encourage states to adopt best practices, with grant funding or enhanced federal matching money. National foundation funding would also be helpful to evaluate and replicate promising outreach and enrollment innovations.

The Massachusetts reform also demonstrates that the ACA may not lead to a reduction in employer-provided coverage, as many have suggested. The individual mandate makes health insurance a more, not less, important employer-provided benefit. The ACA also provides subsidies for small businesses that make coverage available to their employees, while the goal of the exchanges is to make more affordable, stable insurance products available in the small group market. Still, reform will provide strong incentives for employers to shift lower-wage workers to subsidized care through the exchange, where such workers may be fully subsidized. Any such shifts will need to be monitored closely and appropriate corrective action taken.

LESSONS LEARNED

CHIP, HIPAA, and the Massachusetts reform offer many insights and lessons for the implementation of national reform. The remaining analysis applies insight from the examination of federalism across the policy processes in these three cases to the ACA's expansion of Medicaid and the creation of health care exchanges. These changes are estimated to cover 30 million of the nation's uninsured.[12]

Medicaid

The ACA provides significant funding to expand Medicaid for qualified residents with a family income of up to 138 percent of the federal poverty level (FPL).[13] Historically, many of the very poor have not been eligible for Medicaid regardless of their income, particularly single adults or couples without children. This provision will create for the first time a solid health insurance safety net for the vulnerable in the United States. Medicaid is expected to cover 17 million newly insured people under the ACA.[14] The federal government will pay 100 percent of the cost of newly eligible Medicaid beneficiaries and gradually reduce that amount to 90 percent over several years. The

Supreme Court, however, ruled that states do not have to expand Medicaid coverage as required by the ACA, and a number of states have suggested that they may not.[15]

Republican-led states opposed to the ACA have some political and economic calculations to make in the wake of President Obama's reelection. Not expanding Medicaid entails a cost that has primary and secondary effects. Some of the challenge comes because the ACA is funded in part by a reduction in Medicare hospital payments. Hospitals actually agreed to significant cuts because projected revenue from newly insured patients will far exceed those payments. Here is the connection back to Medicaid: states that do not expand Medicaid will experience Medicare cuts and still have to treat a large number of uninsured people for "free." States that do not expand will pay the cost without realizing the full benefits of the reduction in the number of uninsured people. If they do not expand Medicaid, states like Mississippi and Louisiana will in effect subsidize hospitals and uninsured individuals in states like New York, Massachusetts, and California. That certainly will not sit well.

Further, states that do not expand Medicaid leave a lot of federal money on the table. For example, if Texas elects to expand Medicaid, the program is estimated to cover 1.8 million uninsured citizens.[16] Over ten years, the state will need to spend an additional $3.9 billion, a 3.5 percent increase in program costs, but by doing so will capture $952 billion in federal funding.[17] Even by national deficit standards, that is a lot of money. The revenue not only provides coverage for the uninsured but also provides jobs for health care professionals. However, since the Obama administration has a lot riding on state expansion of Medicaid, some states are holding out and trying to cut deals to expand coverage in exchange for increased Medicaid flexibility or even more favorable federal funding arrangements. It is a high-stakes intergovernmental game of "chicken." For comparison, in the past many states said that on principle, they would not take federal economic stimulus money under the Obama administration. But in the end the cash was too hard to resist, and all the states ended up taking stimulus funding. I believe that eventually, due to the power of the hospitals and the lure of federal money, that nearly all the states will participate and end up expanding Medicaid eligibility.

The three cases analyzed here suggest that Medicaid expansion will work. The states have the administrative capacity and expertise to run Medicaid programs. At the federal level, CMS has the operating routines, reporting requirements, and cash incentives to oversee the program. CHIP demonstrated that enhanced federal money leads to greater coverage levels and more consistency in coverage levels among states. CHIP outreach also led to greater coverage in the traditional Medicaid program, for which the states have to pay their traditional, higher share of the costs. From this and the Massachusetts experience, we can anticipate that the individual mandate along with Medicaid expansion will increase enrollment in the traditional Medicaid program. That is great for coverage, but it will also lead to higher-than-anticipated costs for states. In the end, expansion will be less about administrative capacity and more about political will. Health care exchanges will be far more challenging.

Exchanges

Health care exchanges will have a number of functions, including creation of a shopping window for comparing and purchasing health insurance and administration of federal subsidies. Subsidies will be provided through the tax code for people with family incomes from 138 to 400 percent of the federal poverty level. Subsidies will limit the cost of health insurance premiums to between 3.0 and 9.5 percent of income. States will have the option of combining the individual insurance market and the small group market or creating two separate pools. Combining the groups gives the advantage to the individual market because as a group it has higher health care costs and would benefit most from the merger by experiencing lower relative premiums. States that run their own exchanges will also have to choose how active the exchange will be.

Will exchanges look more like the pre-reform system operating in Utah, which had a passive organizing function and includes all current insurance benefit and price variations? Or will they be able to negotiate with and exclude insurance companies from participation, as envisioned by California? Will benefits be uniform? Will a minimum coverage standard be required and, if so, how comprehensive will it be? How will subsidies work? Will they truly make health insurance affordable and the mandate reasonable? All these details will be decided and modified by administrative rules. Then, once the rules are in place, the intergovernmental dynamic will determine how the exchanges affect people and whether they will ultimately succeed or not.

In December 2012, eighteen states indicated that they will develop their own exchanges, eight or nine states indicated that they will create hybrid exchanges in partnership with the federal government, and the rest will likely have largely federally run exchanges.[18] Republican governors and state legislatures are torn between the belief that Obamacare is so objectionable that they should not dignify it by engaging with the federal government and the equally appalling idea of letting the federal government come in and run the exchanges. Conservative leaders in Washington are largely for disengagement, but some Republican governors have had second thoughts. "Our options have come down to this: Do nothing and be at the federal government's mercy in how that exchange is designed and run, or take a seat at the table and play the cards we've been dealt," said the governor of Idaho, C. L. "Butch" Otter. "I cannot willingly surrender a role for Idaho in determining the impact on our own citizens and businesses."[19]

If a state fails to operate a health care exchange under the ACA, the federal government is to come in and do it. Once again, as with HIPAA, the federal government does not have the resources or technical expertise needed to carry out its threat and that fact empowers the states. The first regulations on exchanges gave the states considerable flexibility, including the same time extensions for "effort" that were seen with HIPAA.[20] Deadlines for states to submit plans for creating exchanges continually shifted, and another option for creating a hybrid federal-state exchange was offered. Sandy Praeger, the Kansas insurance commissioner and a National Association of Insurance Commissioners (NAIC) official, confirmed that the federal government bent over backward to accommodate the states, urging them to create their own exchanges.[21] Should such flexibility devolve into "anything goes" exchanges, the law could be weakened and coverage and cost-containment goals could become elusive.

Health care exchanges do not come online until 2014, but systems must be in place prior to the deadline. The more engaged states are in the process of creating exchanges, the more invested they will be in the process and the greater the likelihood that reform will have a chance to succeed. States will need flexibility in establishing exchanges because of the wide diversity in health insurance markets. The challenge will be far greater than in Massachusetts because most states do not have the building blocks and base systems that the Bay State developed over time. During the initial stage of rulemaking, the federal government should collaborate as much as possible with the states. Doing so will acknowledge state variations and perhaps increase the states' acceptance of and participation in the process. Informal channels also need to be established to ensure that federal guidelines mesh with established state insurance baselines and capacity.

CMS should refrain from its overreliance on prescriptive directors, who so enraged the states during CHIP formal rulemaking. To succeed, federal officials need to recognize how last-minute rule changes and adjustments often require costly changes to state training, enrollment, and health information systems. States often view communication with CMS as a one-way black hole. Federal administrators need to provide feedback on data provided by the states to demonstrate the value of the information.

The best model is the early stages of CHIP collaboration, when federal and state officials cooperated to get the program up and running. Federal domination of and federal capitulation to the states may be equally damaging. Federal officials need to hold the states accountable for what is essential while being flexible on the means and timetables. For example, a uniform benefits package is necessary within an exchange in order to make apples-to-apples comparisons of health plans, but permitting differences in benefits packages between states will allow for building on the existing base health care offering in individual states. Enhancing flexibility even at the cost of national uniformity may be essential to the ACA's survival.

However, operating health exchanges is far different from administering CHIP and Medicaid. CMS does not have the existing systems, resources, or expertise to regulate insurance at the state level; HIPAA regulation did not institutionalize such expertise within CMS. Even worse, adopting the Medicare and Medicaid regulatory culture may restrict the state flexibility necessary to make exchanges function well.

An Independent Center for State-Based Exchanges

The Centers for Medicare and Medicaid Services may not be the best agency to oversee health care exchanges. The CHIP case suggests that CMS has the culture, expertise, routines, and resources to oversee the ACA's Medicaid expansion. The HIPAA case suggests that the agency does not have similar expertise and systems in the area of insurance regulation. CMS is likely to take one of two paths, both of which are suboptimal. First, as with CHIP, CMS may start out in collaboration with the states but ultimately move to a top-down regulatory regime similar to Medicare and Medicaid. But without the needed expertise and understanding of state-based insurance markets, that could lead to inefficiency and state frustration. Second, CMS could lower the bar regarding what an acceptable state health exchange is and, as it did with HIPAA, contract out as much of the oversight and technical assistance responsibility as possible and devolve power and responsibility to the states, with limited information and oversight. The consequences will be far reaching: exchanges that do or do not meet the goals of the legislation. Of course, CMS could change its culture by moving to a more collaborative model, hire staff with the requisite expertise, and acquire the needed resources, but that would be difficult. It would take a considerable increase in resources for administration, which Congress would not be likely to approve.

An alternative is to take responsibility for health care exchanges out of CMS and create an independent "Center for State-Based Health Exchanges."

This independent authority could grow out of a bipartisan effort to broaden support for reform and significantly increase the participation of the states. Its impact might be enhanced by the appointment of a Republican as its first administrator. It could be staffed by the current team at CMS, with additional people from the Department of Labor, the Department of the Treasury, insurance experts from the states, and industry. An independent authority holds the possibility of further calming the political hostility at the legislative level and moves the debate toward collaborative regulations and implementation. It increases the chances of finding the intergovernmental sweet spot, providing flexibility for innovation between bounded corridors that ensure program integrity and moving toward fulfilling the ACA's coverage expansion and cost-containment goals.

Away from CMS, the new center could create a culture of partnership and cooperation with states that would significantly increase the possibility of successful implementation. The center could provide states with technical assistance and funding and publicize successful models. It could work closely with the states and associations such as the National Governors Association (NGA), the National Conference of State Legislatures (NCSL), and the National Academy for State Health Policy (NASHP) to elicit state input and help identify and disseminate best practices. When states see other states operating successful exchanges, they will not want to be left out. The key will be to work with early adopters. To its credit, CMS is funding advanced health information technology and eligibility and enrollment systems in several states to serve as models for the rest, but the timeframes here are tight and connecting state, health care exchange, and federal databases is a monumental undertaking.[22] CMS has identified states with advance enrollment systems that could be used by exchanges and has supported the adoption of software and technical assistance that will help all states.

The new center could also work more closely with the Small Business Administration and do a better job of engaging this set of stakeholders, who historically have not been engaged by CMS. Small business opposition could undermine reform by reinforcing opponents' characterization of reform on talk radio and the like as a case of "big government" killing jobs. The key to engaging these stakeholders is to understand and work toward meeting their goals: ease of administration and predictable, lower-cost insurance options for workers and families. If small business owners can talk with friends and business associates about the tangible benefits of health care exchanges, health care reform will be on the right track. The key will be to foster collaboration, align incentives, share information, and document and publicize successes.

A Final Word on Federalism

The analysis of federalism in practice presented in this volume reveals a complex intergovernmental dynamic that unfolds across the policy process. Old studies of intergovernmental relations that focused disproportionately on the legislative process provide limited insight into where and how critical policy decisions are made. More attention needs to be placed on the study of the rulemaking and implementation process and the factors that influence the intergovernmental dance, such as administrative capacity, routines, expertise, resources, reporting requirements, and commitment to achieving program goals. Insights into those factors can help scholars and political scientists to better understand policy formation and implementation and can be used to help advocates germinate and develop policy at the state level, which could benefit the nation.

This analysis can be used to help shape intergovernmental systems that combine national accountability with state responsiveness to local conditions. The account given here of how American federalism plays out in practice is complex and difficult to explain over a beer, but opening this black box is essential to understanding how and by whom or what programs like the ACA are influenced, shaped, and implemented and how they ultimately impact people.

NOTES

CHAPTER 1

1. Paul Starr, *The Social Transformation of American Medicine* (New York: Basic Books, 1982); David Blumenthal and James A. Morone, *The Heart of Power: Health and Politics in the Oval Office* (University of California Press, 2009).

2. John E. McDonough, *Inside National Health Care Reform* (University of California Press, 2011).

3. Sidney Milkis, *The President and the Parties: The Transformation of the American Party System since the New Deal* (Oxford University Press, 1993).

4. Timothy Conlan, *From New Federalism to Devolution: Twenty-Five Years of Intergovernmental Reform* (Brookings, 1998).

5. *National Federation of Independent Businesses* v. *Sebelius*, Sup. Ct. Dkt, No. 11-393 (U.S. 6/28/12).

6. Kaiser Family Foundation, *Focus on Health Reform*, "Establishing Health Insurance Exchanges: An Overview of State Efforts," August 2012 (www.kff.org/healthreform/upload/8213-2.pdf).

7. Kaiser Family Foundation, *Policy Insights*, "Posts Tagged Public Opinion," August 2012 (http://healthreform.kff.org/public-opinion.aspx).

8. Testimony of Alan Weil, executive director, National Academy for State Health Policy, California Legislature, Joint Hearing of the Senate Health Committee and Assembly Health Committee, "Implementation of Federal Health Care Reform," May 12, 2010 (http://nashp.org/sites/default/files/Weil_California_Health_Hearing_Testimony_As_Delivered_May_2010.pdf.)

9. Thomas J. Anton, "New Federalism and Intergovernmental Relationships: The Implications for Health Policy," *Journal of Health Policy Politics and Law* 22, no. 3 (June 1997).

10. D. S. Wright, *Understanding Intergovernmental Relations* (Pacific Grove, Calif.: Brooks/Cole Publishing 1988).

11. Jill Quadagno, *The Color of Welfare: How Racism Undermined the War on Poverty* (Oxford University Press, 1994).

12. Lyndon B. Johnson, University of Michigan Commencement Address (Great Society speech), May 22, 1964 (www.michigandaily.com/content/president-lyndon-b-johnsons-commencement-address-university-michigan-may-22-1964-0).

13. Paul L. Posner, *The Politics of Unfunded Mandates* (Georgetown University Press, 1998).

14. Wright, *Understanding Intergovernmental Relations*; L. J. O'Toole Jr. *American Intergovernmental Relations* (Washington, D.C.: CQ Press, 1985).

15. Robert Rich and William White. *Health Policy, Federalism, and the American States* (Washington: Urban Institute Press, 1996).

16. R. P. Nathan, "The Role of States in American Federalism," in *The State of the States*, 2nd ed., edited by C. E. Van Horn (Washington, D.C.: CQ Press, 1993), pp. 15–30.

17. Paul E. Peterson, *The Price of Federalism* (Brookings, 1995).

18. Michael Greve, *Real Federalism: Why It Matters, How It Could Happen* (Washington: American Enterprise Institute, 1999).

19. Starr, *The Social Transformation of American Medicine.*

20. Paul E. Peterson, Barry G. Rabe, Kenneth K. Wong, *When Federalism Works* (Brookings, 1986).

21. See Timothy Conlan and John Dinan, "Federalism, the Bush Administration, and the Transformation of American Conservatism," *Publius* 37, no. 3 (2007), pp. 279–303; Shama Gamkhar and J. Mitch Pickerill, "The State of American Federalism 2011–2012: A Fend for Yourself and Activist Form of Bottom-Up Federalism," *Publius* (July 3, 2012) (http://publius.oxfordjournals.org/content/early/2012/07/02/publius.pjs027.full).

22. Conlan, *From New Federalism to Devolution*, p. 1.

23. Ibid.

24. Richard P. Nathan, "Updating Theories of Federalism," in *Intergovernmental Management for the Twenty-First Century*, edited by Timothy Conlan and Paul L. Posner (Brookings, 2008), p. 18.

25. William West, "Special Report: Administrative Rulemaking: An Old and Emerging Literature," *Public Administration Review* 65, no. 6 (November-December 2005), pp. 655–68.

26. Marissa Martino Golden, "Interest Groups in the Rule-Making Process: Who Participates? Whose Voices Get Heard?" *Journal of Public Administration Research and Theory*, April 1, 1998.

27. Theodore R. Marmor, *The Politics of Medicare*, 2nd ed. (Hawthorne, N.Y.: Aldine de Gruyter, 2000).

28. Nathan, "Updating Theories of Federalism."

CHAPTER 2

1. Kaiser Commission on Medicaid and the Uninsured, "Medicaid Financing: An Overview of the Federal Medicaid Matching Rate (FMAP)" (September 2012) (www.kff.org/medicaid/upload/8352.pdf).

2. Personal communication, Chris Jennings, senior White House adviser, October 13, 2000.

3. News conference with Senate minority leader Tom Daschle (D-S.D.) and House minority leader Richard Gephardt (D-Mo.), "Adding Children's Health Insurance and Campaign Finance Reform to the 105th Congress' Legislative Agenda," Washington, February 26, 1997 (http://collections.mohistory.org/cdm/Text:5475).

4. Opening statement of Representative Bill Thomas (R-Calif.), *Children's Access to Health Coverage: Hearing before the Subcommittee on Health of the Committee on Ways and Means, House of Representatives*, 105 Cong., 1 sess., April 8, 1997 (www.gpo.gov/fdsys/pkg/CHRG-105hhrg52730/pdf/CHRG-105hhrg52730.pdf).

5. Statement of Senator Don Nickles (R-Okla.), *Increasing Children's Access to Health Care: Hearing before the Committee on Finance, U.S. Senate*, 105 Cong., 1 sess., April 30, 1997 (http://catalog.hathitrust.org/Record/007607885).

6. Statement of Representative Sam Johnson (R-Tex.), *Children's Access to Health Coverage*.

7. Alan Weil, "The New Children's Health Insurance Program: Should States Expand Medicaid?" New Federalism Program Issues and Options for States, Series A, No. A-13 (Washington: Urban Institute, October 1997).

8. Catherine Hoffman and Alan Schlobohm, *Uninsured in America: A Chart Book of the Kaiser Commission on Medicaid and the Uninsured*, 2nd ed. (Washington: Kaiser Commission on Medicaid and the Uninsured, March 2000).

9. Eileen R. Ellis and Vernon K. Smith, "Medicaid Enrollment in 21 States: June 1997" (Washington: Kaiser Commission on Medicaid and the Uninsured, April 2000) (www.kff.org/content/2000/20000412a/pub2190.pdf.)

10. Testimony of Senator Bob Graham (D-Fla.), *Increasing Children's Access to Health Care*.

11. Testimony of Rose Naff, Florida Health Kids Program, *Increasing Children's Access to Health Care*.

12. Ibid.

13. Ellis and Smith, "Medicaid Enrollment in 21 States: June 1997."

14. Hoffman and Schlobohm, *Uninsured in America*.

15. Ibid.

16. Statement of Secretary of Health and Human Services Donna Shalala, *Improving the Health Status of Children: Hearing of the Committee on Labor and Human Resources, U.S. Senate*, 105 Cong., 1 sess., April 18, 1997 (http://catalog.hathitrust.org/Record/003482931).

17. Personal communication, senior Democratic congressional staff member (2000).

18. Personal communication, Laurie Rubiner, former legislative aide to Senator John Chafee (R-R.I.), June 27, 2000.

19. Personal communication, Charles N. Kahn III, president, National Health Insurance Association of America, and former staff director, Committee on Ways and Means, U.S. House of Representatives, June 29, 2000.

20. Representative Sherrod Brown (D-Ohio), the ranking member on the Subcommittee on Health, House Commerce Committee, offered this substitute amendment.

21. Representative Jim Greenwood (R-Pa.), statement, *Congressional Record,* June 25, 1997, p. H4572.

22. Representative Sherrod Brown (D-Ohio), quoted in *Congressional Quarterly Almanac* (Washington: Congressional Quarterly, 1997), pp. 6–7.

23. Representative Patsy Mink (D-Hi.) statement, *Congressional Record,* June 25, 1997, p. H4575.

24. Personal communication, senior administration official (2000).

25. "Big Medicare, Medicaid Changes Enacted in the Budget Bills," *Congressional Quarterly Almanac* (Washington: Congressional Quarterly, 1997).

26. Robert Pear, "Senate Panel Rebuffs Clinton on Child Health Plan," *New York Times,* June 18, 1997, p. 22.

27. Personal communication, Laurie Rubiner.

28. Ibid.

29. Pear, "Senate Panel Rebuffs Clinton on Child Health Plan."

30. Senator Tom Daschle (D-S.D.) testified at *Increasing Children's Access to Health Care,* April 30, 1997, that "Senator Hatch, in particular, has shown real leadership on this issue—and taken some heat for it. It's a sad commentary on this Congress that supporting a modest children's health bill can get you denounced in your own caucus."

31. Senator Edward Kennedy, statement, *Congressional Record,* May 21, 1997, p. S4815.

32. Ibid., p. S4816.

33. Recorded vote, *Congressional Record,* May 21, 1997, p. S4827.

34. Senator Orrin Hatch (R-Utah), statement, *Congressional Record,* May 21, 1997, p. S4827.

35. Personal communication, senior Democratic congressional staff member (2000).

36. Ibid.

37. Personal communication, Shelly Gehshan, senior staff person, National Council of State Legislatures (NCSL), May 24, 2000.

38. Personal communication, Laurie Rubiner.

39. Personal communication, Dean Rosen, chief counsel, National Health Insurance Association of America, and former senior staff counsel to Senator Nancy Kassebaum, June 29, 2000.

40. Personal communication, Joan Henneberry, National Governors Association, June 30, 2000.

41. National Governors Association, "Governors Urge Conferees to Enact Legislation That Will Help, Not Hinder," news release (Washington: July 7, 1997).

42. Ibid.

43. Personal communication, senior administration official (2000).

44. The National Governors Association adopted these comments on children's health at the association's 2000 annual meeting, Las Vegas, Nevada, July 27–30, 2000.

45. Personal communication, senior administration official.

46. Personal communication, Chris Jennings.

47. *Title XXI: State Children's Health Insurance Program*, appears in the U.S. Code as §§1397aa-1397mm, subchapter XXI, chapter 7, title 42. This reference is to sec. 2105 (c)(7) and sec. 2109.

48. Title XXI, sec. 2103.

49. Deborah Stone, *Policy Paradox: The Art of Political Decision Making* (New York: W.W. Norton, 1997).

CHAPTER 3

1. Andrew Siddons, "Debates Put Focus on Romney's 'Day 1' Pledges," *New York Times*, October 22, 1912 (http://thecaucus.blogs.nytimes.com/2012/10/22/debates-put-focus-on-romneys-day-1-pledges/).

2. "State Child Health: Implementing Regulations for the State Children's Health Insurance Program: Proposed Rule," *Federal Register* 64, no. 215 (November 8, 1999), p. 60883 (www.gpo.gov/fdsys/pkg/FR-1999-11-08/html/99-28693.htm).

3. The rulemaking procedures are outlined in the Administrative Procedure Act, Title 5, U.S. Code, chapter 5, sections 511–599.

4. Personal communication, Debbie Chang, Maryland Medicaid director and former senior official in charge of CHIP rulemaking at CMS, July 19, 2000.

5. For example, the October 18, 1999, "Dear State Health Official" letter provides information on school-based enrollment. The September 10 and November 23, 1998, letters provided information on states that had been successful in implementing joint CHIP-Medicaid applications.

6. Personal communications, Bruce Bullen, former director of the National Association of Medicaid Directors and former Massachusetts Medicaid director, November 30, 2000; personal communications, Christie Ferguson, former director Rhode Island Health and Human Services, December 5, 2000.

7. Personal communication, Debbie Chang.

8. Personal communication, Shelly Gehshan, National Conference of State Legislatures, May 24, 2000.

9. House Committee on Commerce, "State Children's Health Insurance Program (S-CHIP) Implementation Guide" (Washington: November 1997).

10. Personal communication, Debbie Chang.

11. Ibid.

12. Personal communication, Cherilyn Cepriano, National Governors Association, Health Division, June 30, 2000.

13. Comments from the State of Florida on the proposed CHIP rule (Baltimore: CMS, January 5, 2000).

14. Comments from the Commonwealth of Virginia on the proposed CHIP rule (Baltimore: CMS, January 6, 2000).

15. Presidential Executive Order on Federalism, no.13132 (Washington: August 10, 1999).

16. Personal communication, Cherilyn Cepriano.

17. Comments from the National Conference of State Legislatures on the proposed CHIP rule (Baltimore: CMS, January 7, 2000).

18. CMS, "State Children's Health Insurance Series of Question and Answers," question number 44 (Baltimore: CMS, 2000).

19. CMS, "State Children's Health Insurance Series of Question and Answers," question number 46.

20. *Federal Register*, p. 60900.

21. Ibid., p. 60898.

22. CMS, "State Children's Health Insurance Series of Questions and Answers," Question number 14 (a) (2000).

23. *Federal Register*, p. 60902.

24. Ibid., p. 60894.

25. Ibid., p. 60907.

26. Ibid., p. 60908

27. Comments from the Commonwealth of Massachusetts on the proposed CHIP rule (Baltimore: CMS, January 1, 2000).

28. *Federal Register*, p. 60906.

29. Ibid., p. 60915.

30. Ibid., p. 60906.

31. Comments from the State of California on the proposed CHIP rule (Baltimore: CMS, January 6, 2000).

32. Comments from the State of Kentucky on the proposed CHIP rule (Baltimore: CMS, January 5, 2000).

33. *Federal Register*, p. 60909.

34. Ibid., p. 60891.

35. Ibid., p. 60916.

36. "Dear State Health Official" letter from Sally K. Richardson, director, CMS (September 10, 1998).

37. "Dear State Health Official" letter from Sally K. Richardson, director, CMS (November 23, 1998).

38. Comments from the State of Utah on the proposed CHIP rule (Baltimore: CMS, January 6, 2000).

39. Comments from the State of Alabama on the proposed CHIP rule (Baltimore: CMS, January 6, 2000).

40. Comments from various advocates on the proposed CHIP rule (Baltimore: CMS, 2000).

41. Ibid.

42. *Federal Register*, pp. 60928–30.

43. Ibid.

44. Personal communication, Cherilyn Cepriano.

45. *Federal Register*, p. 60926.

46. Ibid., p. 60911.

47. Comments from various advocates on the proposed CHIP rule.

CHAPTER 4

1. Vernon K. Smith, David M. Rousseau, and Jocelyn A. Guyer, "CHIP Program Enrollment: 2000" (Washington: Kaiser Commission on Medicaid and the Uninsured, September 2001), p. 17.

2. John Iglehart, "The Battle over SCHIP," *New England Journal of Medicine* 357, no. 10 (September 6, 2007), p. 957.

3. "Testimony on the Children's Health Insurance Program by Nancy-Ann DeParle, Administrator, Health Care Financing Administration, U.S. Department of Health and Human Services before the Senate Finance Committee," April 29, 1999 (www.dhhs.gov/asl/testify/t990429a.html).

4. Judith Havemann, "Child Health Program Gets Off to a Slow Start; Only 828,000 Uninsured Now Enrolled," *Washington Post*, April 13, 1999, p. A 19.

5. Department of Health and Human Services, "The State Children's Health Insurance Program Annual Enrollment Report, October, 1998 through September 1999" (Washington: 2000).

6. Robert Pear, "40 States Forfeit Health Care Funds for Poor Children," *New York Times*, September 24, 2000, p. A1.

7. Havemann, "Child Health Program Gets Off to a Slow Start."

8. L.M. Feder, M. Panagides-Busch, R. Schulzinger, "The Child Health Insurance Program: Early Implementation in Six States," prepared for the U.S . Department of Health and Human Services (Washington: American Institute for Research, July 1999).

9. F. Ullman, B. Bruen, and J. Holahan, "The States' Children's Health Insurance Program: A Look at the Numbers" (Washington: Urban Institute, March 1998).

10. Ibid.

11. "Children's Health Insurance Program: State Implementation Approaches Are Evolving," U.S. General Accounting Office Report, GAO/HEHS-99-65 (Washington: May 1999), p. 12.

12. Robert Pear, "Feds Holding Unspent Money in Kids' Health Insurance Plan; Mixed Signals from Agents Hindered States from Using Full Allotment, Officials Say," *Milwaukee Journal-Sentinel*, September 24, 2000, p. 18 A.

13. M. Bombardieri, "Windfall to Boost Mass Child Health," *Boston Globe,* September 25, 2000, p. A1.

14. Ibid.

15. Pear, "Feds Holding Unspent Money in Kids' Health Insurance Plan."

16. Pear, "40 States Forfeit Health Care Funds for Poor Children."

17. Ibid.

18. Children's Defense Fund, "All Over the Map: A Progress Report on the State Children's Health Insurance Program (CHIP)" (Washington: July 2000), p. 20.

19. Personal communications, senior Democratic legislative staff member (2000).

20. Personal communications, Christie Ferguson, former director of Rhode Island Health and Human Services, December 5, 2000.

21. Smith, Rousseau, and Guyer, "CHIP Program Enrollment: 2000."

22. Ullman, Bruen and Holahan, "The States' Children's Health Insurance Program."

23. Information on governors' support comes from Alan Weil, Urban Institute director, "Federalism: The Role of States in Health Policy in the Bush Administration," Assessing the New Federalism Program Lecture, Waltham, Massachusetts, January 29, 2001; personal communications, Chris Jennings, senior White House health policy adviser, October 13, 2000. Jennings stated that even conservative Senator Roth (R-Del.) took credit for helping create the CHIP program.

24. Ian Hill, "Charting New Courses for Children's Health Insurance," *Policy and Practice: The Journal of the American Public Human Services Association* 58, no. 4 (December 2000), pp. 30–38.

25. Personal communication, Debbie Chang, Maryland Medicaid director and former senior official in charge of CHIP rulemaking at CMS, July 19, 2000.

26. Ibid.

27. Ibid.

28. Children's Defense Fund, "All Over the Map."

29. "Children's Health Insurance Program: State Implementation Approaches Are Evolving."

30. Ibid.

31. Children's Defense Fund, "All Over the Map."

32. Public Law 106-113.

33. Hill, "Charting New Courses for Children's Health Insurance."

34. Children's Defense Fund, "All Over the Map."

35. "Children's Health Insurance Program: State Implementation Approaches Are Evolving."

36. Ibid., p. 2.

37. Ibid., p. 48.

38. Ibid.

39. Ibid.

40. Ibid.

41. Ibid., p. 35.

42. Sarah Rosenbaum, A. Markus, and D. Roby, "An Analysis of Implementation Issues Relating to CHIP Cost-Sharing Provisions for Certain Targeted Low-Income Children" (Washington: Health Care Financing Administration and the Health Resources and Services Administration, June 1999).

43. "United States General Accounting Office Report to Congressional Committees" (1999).

44. Hill, "Charting New Courses for Children's Health Insurance.".

45. Personal communication, Debbie Chang.

46. Personal communication, Bruce Bullen, former director of the National Association of Medicaid Directors and former Massachusetts Medicaid director, November 30, 2000.

47. Personal communication, Debbie Chang.

48. Personal communication, Bruce Bullen. Bullen noted that past CMS regulations tried to standardize the way that CMS deals with Section 1115 waivers. This striving toward uniformity may be a way to cope with staff shortages and the policy goals of interest groups, the administration, and members of Congress, but it contravenes the very concept of waivers, which by definition are unique approaches to meeting program goals.

49. Ibid.

50. Ibid.

51. Ibid.

52. Personal communications, Christie Ferguson.

53. Personal communications, Joan Heneberry, National Governors Association, June 30, 2000.

54. Personal communications, Debbie Chang.

55. Personal communications, Shelly Geshan, National Council State Legislators, May 24, 2000.

56. Personal communications, Debbie Chang.

57. Personal communications, Bruce Bullen.

58. Now CMS is using the Massachusetts employer subsidy program as an example of innovation.

59. Pear, "Feds Holding Unspent Money in Kids' Health Insurance Plan."

60. Personal communications, Christie Ferguson.

CHAPTER 5

1. "Health Insurance Standards: New Federal Law Creates Challenges for Consumers, Insurers, Regulators," GAO HEHS-98-67 (U.S. General Accounting Office, February 25, 1998).

2. Personal communication, Dean Rosen, chief counsel, National Health Insurance Association of America, and former senior staff counsel to Senator Nancy Kassebaum, June 29, 2000.

3. Ibid.

4. Personal communication, Kala Ladenheim, National Conference of State Legislatures, May 24, 2000.

5. Liberal supporters of the bill wanted to credit Senator Kennedy. Conservatives, including Newt Gingrich, who opposed the bill, referred to it as Kennedy-Kassebaum, using Kennedy as a pejorative symbol of "big liberal government."

6. Senator Edward Kennedy (D-Mass.), Statement, *Congressional Record*, April 18, 1996, p. S.3513.

7. Senator Jay Rockefeller (D-W.Va.), Statement, *Congressional Record*, April 18, 1996, p. S.3514.

8. Senator Jim Jeffords (R-Vt.), Statement, *Congressional Record*, April 18, 1996, p. S.3519.

9. Senator Bill Roth (R-Del.), Statement, *Congressional Record*, April 18, 1996, p. S. 3545.

10. Senator Paul Wellstone (D-Minn.), Statement, *Congressional Record*, April 18, 1996, p. S. 3519.

11. Paul Fronstin and Sara R. Collins, "Early Experience with High-Deductible and Consumer-Driven Health Plans: Findings from the EBRI/Commonwealth Fund Consumerism in Health Care Survey" (New York: Commonwealth Fund, December 2005).

12. Senator Nancy Kassebaum (R-Kans.), Statement, *Congressional Record*, April 18, 1996, p. S. 3530.

13. Senator Jim Jeffords, Statement, *Congressional Record*.

14. Representative Marge Roukema was a moderate Republican from New Jersey.

15. Speaker Newt Gingrich. (R-Ga.), Statement, *Congressional Record*, August 1, 1996, p. H3135.

16. Representative Denis Hastert (R-Ill.), Statement, *Congressional Record*, August 1, 1996, p. H3096.

17. "House Passes Republican Health Reform Bill, 267-151." *Congress Daily*, March 29, 1996.

18. Speaker Newt Gingrich, Statement, *Congressional Record*.

19. Ed Gillespie, Dick Armey, and Bob Schellhas, *Contract with America* (New York: Crown Publishing Group, December 26, 1994).

20. Representative Jack Kingston (R-Ga.), Statement, *Congressional Record*, August 1, 1996, p. H3095.

21. Speaker Newt Gingrich, Statement, *Congressional Record*.

22. Representative Harris Fawell (R-Ill.), Statement, *Congressional Record*, August 1, 1996, p. H3101.

23 Representative Ben Cardin (D-Md), Statement, *Congressional Record*, August 1, 1996, p. H3085.

24. Ibid.

25. "GOP Predicts Health Bill 'Love Fest'; Dems See War," *Congress Daily*, March 25, 1996.

26. Representative Peter DeFazio (D-Ore.), Statement, *Congressional Record,* August 1, 1996, p. H3107.

27. Tom Bliley (R-Va.), Statement, *Congressional Record,* August 1, 1996, p. H3090.

28. Personal communication, Charles N. Kahn III, president, National Health Insurance Association of America and former staff director, House of Representatives Committee on Ways and Means, June 29, 2000.

29. Letter from the National Association of Insurance Commissioners to Speaker Gingrich, March 28, 1996, referring to Title I, Subtitle D, Section 192, of House bill H.R.3103. Reprinted in the *Congressional Record,* August 1, 1996, p. H3099.

30. Personal communication, Charles N. Kahn III.

31. Ibid.

32. Personal communication, Dean Rosen.

33. Ibid.

34. Ibid.

35. Personal communication, Kala Ladenheim.

36. Ibid.

37. Personal communication, Nicole Tapay, CMS senior staff, formerly with the National Association of Insurance Commissioners, June 28, 2000.

38. Personal communication, Dean Rosen.

39. Ibid.

40. Ibid.

41. Personal communication, Nicole Tapay.

42. Ibid.

43. Joy Wilson, "NCSL Health Committee Bill Summary: The Health Insurance Portability and Accountability Act of 1996" (Washington: National Conference of State Legislatures, August 13, 1996).

44. Health Insurance Portability and Accountability Act of 1996, P. L. 104-191, sec. 701(a) (1).

45. Personal communication, Dean Rosen.

46. Personal communication, Charles N. Kahn III.

47. Health Insurance Portability and Accountability Act of 1996, sec. 2741 (a)(2).

48. Ibid., sec. 2772 (b)(2)(B).

CHAPTER 6

1. "Patient Protection and Affordable Care Act; Establishment of Exchanges and Qualified Health Plans; Proposed Rule," *Federal Register* 75, no. 136 (July 15, 2011).

2. Testimony of David H. Ennis, Delaware House of Representatives, on behalf of the National Conference of State Legislatures, *Health Insurance Portability and Accountability Act 1996: Hearing before the Labor and Human Resources Committee, U.S. Senate,* 105 Cong., 1 sess., February 11, 1997.

3. States whose legislatures did not meet within twelve months of HIPAA's enactment had until July 1, 1998.

4. The authority to issue rules in this form comes from the Public Health Service Act (42 U.S.C., sec. 300gg-92), ERISA (29 U.S.C., sec. 1191c), the Internal Revenue Code (26 U.S.C., sec. 9833), and the Administrative Procedure Act (5 U.S.C., sec. 553b).

5. CMS administers the Medicare program through contracts with insurance intermediaries and carriers that process claims or bills from hospitals, doctors, and other authorized Medicare providers. This is not direct regulation.

6. "Health Insurance Portability for Group Health Plans; Interim Rules and Proposed Rule," *Federal Register* 62, no. 67 (April 8, 1997), p. 16895.

7. Testimony of Chris Petersen, vice president, Health Insurance Association of America, *Health Insurance Portability and Accountability Act of 1996*.

8. "Health Insurance Portability for Group Health Plans; Interim Rules and Proposed Rule," p. 16913.

9. Testimony of Bruce Vladeck, administrator of the Health Care Financing Administration, *Health Insurance Portability and Accountability Act of 1996* (www.hhs.gov/asl/testify/t970211a.html).

10. Ibid.

11. Discussion between Senator Mike Enzi (R-Wyo.) and Joy Wilson, National Conference of State Legislatures, *Health Insurance Portability and Accountability Act of 1996*.

12. Testimony of Bruce Vladeck, *Health Insurance Portability and Accountability Act of 1996*.

13. Response of Joy Wilson, National Conference of State Legislatures, to a question by Senator Jim Jeffords (R-Vt.), *Health Insurance Portability and Accountability Act of 1996*.

14. Response of Josephine Musser, president of the National Association of Insurance Commissioners, to a question by Senator Jim Jeffords (R-Vt.), *Health Insurance Portability and Accountability Act of 1996*.

15. "Health Insurance Standards: New Federal Law Creates Challenges for Consumers, Insurers, Regulators," GAO/HEHS-98-67 (General Accounting Office, February 1998) (www.gao.gov/assets/230/225350.pdf).

16. Testimony of Bruce Vladeck, *Health Insurance Portability and Accountability Act of 1996*.

17. Ibid.

18. Testimony of Chris Peterson, *Health Insurance Portability and Accountability Act of 1996*.

19. Testimony of Bruce Vladeck, *Health Insurance Portability and Accountability Act of 1996*.

20. Personal communication, Bruce Bullen, former director of the National Association of Medicaid Directors and former Massachusetts Medicaid director, November 30, 2000.

21. Testimony of Terry Humo, assistant vice president, Sedgwick, Nobel, and Lowndes, on behalf of the Association of Private Pension and Welfare Plans, *Health Insurance Portability and Accountability Act of 1996* .

22. Personal communication, Dean Rosen, chief counsel, National Health Insurance Association of America, and former senior staff counsel to Senator Nancy Kassebaum, June 29, 2000.

23. Testimony of Josephine Musser, president of the National Association of Insurance Commissioners, *Health Insurance Portability and Accountability Act of 1996.*

24. Testimony of Gail Shearer, Consumers Union, *Health Insurance Portability and Accountability Act of 1996.*

25. "Health Insurance Portability for Group Health Plans; Interim Rules and Proposed Rule," p. 16908.

26. Ibid., p. 16895.

27. Ibid., p. 16897.

28. "Federal Enforcement in Group and Individual Health Insurance Markets," *Federal Register* 64, no. 161 (August 20, 1999).

29. "Health Insurance Portability for Group Health Plans; Interim Rules and Proposed Rule," p. 16919.

30. Ibid., p. 16914.

31. Ibid., p. 16904.

32. Ibid., p. 16905.

33. Ibid., p. 16913.

34. Ibid. p., 16926.

35. Ibid., p. 16913.

36. Ibid. p. 16986.

37. Ibid., p. 16914.

38. Ibid., p. 16991.

39. Ibid., p. 16916.

40. "Federal Enforcement in Group and Individual Health Insurance Markets," p. 45786.

41. "Health Insurance Portability for Group Health Plans; Interim Rules and Proposed Rule," p. 16991.

42. "Federal Enforcement in Group and Individual Health Insurance Markets," p. 45794.

43. Comments from the National Association of Insurance Commissioners on the HIPAA proposed rule to secretaries Summers (Treasury), Shalala (Health and Human Services), and Herman (Labor) (Baltimore: CMS, January 24, 2000).

44. Comments from the National Association of Insurance Commissioners on the HIPAA proposed rule.

45. Meghan McCarthy, "New Health Exchange Regulations Make Room for Brokers," *National Journal,* March 12, 2012) (www.nationaljournal.com/healthcare/new-health-exchange-regulations-make-room-for-brokers-20120312).

46. Ibid.

CHAPTER 7

1. Stephen H. Long and M. Susan Marquis, "Baseline Information for Evaluating the Implementation of the Health Insurance Portability and Accountability Act of 1996: Final Report," prepared for CMS by the RAND Corporation (Baltimore: October 1998) (http://aspe.hhs.gov/health/reports/hipabase/toc.htm).

2. Personal communication, senior Internal Revenue Service official (2001).

3. Personal communication, senior Department of Labor Official (2000).

4. "Health Insurance Standards: New Federal Law Creates Challenges for Consumers, Insurers, Regulators," GAO/HEHS-98-67 (General Accounting Office, February 1998) (www.gao.gov/assets/230/225350.pdf).

5. CMS is also responsible for ensuring that self-insured state and local government plans meet HIPAA requirements. However, in another twist on federalism, HIPAA permits state and local governments that sponsor self-funded group plans to exempt those plans from all or any part of HIPAA requirements. CMS has taken no action in this area.

6. "Private Health Insurance: HCFA Cautious in Enforcing Federal HIPAA Standards in States Lacking Conforming Laws," GAO/HEHS-98-217R (General Accounting Office, July 22, 1998), p. 3 (www.gao.gov/assets/90/88060.pdf).

7. Ibid.

8. Ibid., p. 16.

9. Testimony on the Health Insurance Portability and Accountability Act by Nancy-Ann Min DeParle, Administrator, Health Care Financing Administration, U.S. Department of Health and Human Services, before the Senate Committee on Labor and Human Resources, March 19, 1998 (www.hhs.gov/asl/testify/t980319d.html).

10. Ibid.

11. "Private Health Insurance: HCFA Cautious in Enforcing Federal HIPAA Standards in States Lacking Conforming Laws," p. 13.

12. Ibid., p.12.

13. "Implementation of HIPAA: Progress Slow in Enforcing Federal Standards in Nonconforming States," GAO/HEHS-00-85 (General Accounting Office, March 31, 2000), p.7 (www.gpo.gov/fdsys/pkg/GAOREPORTS-HEHS-00-85/pdf/GAO REPORTS-HEHS-00-85.pdf).

14. Personal communication, Matt Salvo, director for health legislation, National Governors Association, June 30, 2000.

15. Personal communication, Kala Ladenheim, National Conference of State Legislatures, May 24, 2000.

16 "Implementation of HIPAA: Progress Slow in Enforcing Federal Standards in Nonconforming States," p. 10.

17. Ibid., p. 17.

18. "Private Health Insurance: HCFA Cautious in Enforcing Federal HIPAA Standards in States Lacking Conforming Laws."

19. "Health Insurance Standards: Implications of New Federal Law for Consumers, Insurers, Regulators," GAO/T-HEHS-98-114 (General Accounting Office, March 19, 1998) (www.gpo.gov/fdsys/pkg/GAOREPORTS-T-HEHS-98-114/pdf/GAOREPORTS-T-HEHS-98-114.pdf).

20. "Private Health Insurance: Progress and Challenges in Implementing 1996 Federal Standards," GAO/HEHS-99-100 (General Accounting Office, May 1999) (www.gpo.gov/fdsys/pkg/GAOREPORTS-HEHS-99-100/pdf/GAOREPORTS-HEHS-99-100.pdf).

21. "Private Health Insurance: HCFA Cautious in Enforcing Federal HIPAA Standards in States Lacking Conforming Laws," p. 23.

22. Ibid., p. 13.

23. Ibid., pp. 6–8.

24. Testimony of Jay Angoff, director of the Missouri Department of Insurance, *Implementation of the Health Insurance Portability and Accountability Act: Hearing before the Subcommittee on Health of the Committee on Ways and Means, U.S. House of Representatives*, 105 Cong., 1 sess., September 25, 1997.

25. Karen Pollitz and Nicole Tapay, "The Health Insurance Portability and Accountability Act of 1996: Early Experience with 'New Federalism' in Health Insurance Regulation" (Washington: Institute for Health Care Research and Policy, Georgetown University Medical Center, April 30, 1999).

26. Ibid.

27. "Private Health Insurance: Progress and Challenges in Implementing 1996 Federal Standards," p.23.

28. "Implementation of HIPAA: Progress Slow in Enforcing Federal Standards in Nonconforming States," p. 3.

29. Testimony on the Health Insurance Portability and Accountability Act by Nancy-Ann Min DeParle.

30. "Health Insurance Standards: New Federal Law Creates Challenges for Consumers, Insurers, Regulators," p. 19.

31. "Implementation of HIPAA: Progress Slow in Enforcing Federal Standards in Nonconforming States," p. 11.

32. Personal communication, HIPAA staff member, CMS regional office (2001).

33. Personal communication, Christie Ferguson, director, Rhode Island Health and Human Services, December 5, 2000.

34. "Private Health Insurance: Progress and Challenges in Implementing 1996 Federal Standards," p. 2.

35. Ibid., p. 7.

36. Pollitz and Tapay, "The Health Insurance Portability and Accountability Act of 1996," p. 20.

37. Ibid., p. 8.

38. "Private Health Insurance: HCFA Cautious in Enforcing Federal HIPAA Standards in States Lacking Conforming Laws," p. 23.

39. Pollitz and Tapay, "The Health Insurance Portability and Accountability Act of 1996," p. 10.

40. Ibid.

41. Testimony on the Health Insurance Portability and Accountability Act of 1996 by Alessandro A. Iuppa, Commissioner of Insurance for the State of Maine, on behalf of the National Association of Insurance Commissioners, before the Senate Committee on Labor and Human Resources, March 19, 1998.

42. Ibid.

43. "Private Health Insurance: HCFA Cautious in Enforcing Federal HIPAA Standards in States Lacking Conforming Laws."

44. Ibid., p. 11.

45. J. Gabel and others, "Health Benefits of Small Employers in 1998" (Washington: Henry J. Kaiser Family Foundation, February 1999).

46. Long and Marquis, "Baseline Information for Evaluating the Implementation of the Health Insurance Portability and Accountability Act of 1996."

47. Pollitz and Tapay, p. 13.

48. Ibid., 12.

49. "Private Health Insurance: HCFA (now CMS) Cautious in Enforcing Federal HIPAA Standards in States Lacking Conforming Laws." GAO Report, p. 14.

50. Pollitz and Tapay, "The Health Insurance Portability and Accountability Act of 1996," p. 13.

51. "Private Health Insurance: HCFA Cautious in Enforcing Federal HIPAA Standards in States Lacking Conforming Laws," p. 14.

52. "Health Insurance Standards: New Federal Law Creates Challenges for Consumers, Insurers, Regulators," p. 2.

53. "Private Health Insurance: Progress and Challenges in Implementing 1996 Federal Standards," p. 12.

54. Statement of Senator Jim Jeffords (R-Vt.) on the Health Insurance Portability and Accountability Act of 1996 before the Senate Committee on Labor and Human Resources, March 19, 1998.

55. "Health Insurance Standards: New Federal Law Creates Challenges for Consumers, Insurers, Regulators," p. 6.

56. "Program Memorandum to State Insurance Commissioners and Insurance Issuers from the Health Care Financing Administration," Transmittal No. 98-01 (Baltimore: March 1998).

57. Testimony on Health Insurance Portability and Accountability Act of 1996 by Alessandro A. Iuppa.

58. "Program Memorandum to State Insurance Commissioners and Insurance Issuers from the Health Care Financing Administration."

59. "Private Health Insurance: HCFA Cautious in Enforcing Federal HIPAA Standards in States Lacking Conforming Laws."

60. Ibid.

61. Pollitz and Tapay, "The Health Insurance Portability and Accountability Act of 1996," p. 11.

62. Dean Rosen, "Basics of Private Health Insurance," Alliance for Health Reform and the Kaiser Foundation, conference and Internet simulcast, Washington, D.C., June 1, 2001.

63. "Private Health Insurance: HCFA Cautious in Enforcing Federal HIPAA Standards in States Lacking Conforming Laws," p. 15.

CHAPTER 8

1. Mitt Romney, "What We've Learned from the Massachusetts Health Plan," *Wall Street Journal,* July 12, 2008.

2. Sharon K. Long, "What Is the Evidence on Health Reform in Massachusetts and How Might the Lessons from Massachusetts Apply to National Health Reform?" (Robert Wood Johnson Foundation and the Urban Institute, June 2011) (www.urban.org/uploadedpdf/412118-massachusetts-national-health-reform.pdf).

3. Sharon K. Long and Karen Stockley, "Health Insurance Reform in Massachusetts: An Update as of Fall 2009" (Boston: Blue Cross Blue Shield of Massachusetts Foundation, 2010) (http://bluecrossmafoundation.org/sites/default/files/MHRS%20Report%20Aug24.pdf bluecrossfoundation.org).

4. Sharon K. Long and Karen Stockley, "Sustaining Health Reform in a Recession: An Update on Massachusetts as of Fall 2009," *Health Affairs* 29, no. 6 (2010), pp. 1234–41.

5. Long and Stockley, "Health Insurance Reform in Massachusetts: An Update as of Fall 2009."

6. Massachusetts Taxpayers Foundation, "Massachusetts Health Reform: The Myth of Uncontrolled Costs" (Boston, 2009).

7. John E. McDonough and others, "The Third Wave of Massachusetts Health Care Access Reform," *Health Affairs* (September 2006), p. 421 (http://content.healthaffairs.org/content/25/6/w420.abstract).

8. For more details about the Medicaid program see "Medicaid: A Primer," Kaiser Family Foundation, 2011 (www.kff.org/medicaid/upload/7334-04.pdf)

9. Stephanie Anthony, Robert Seifert, and Jean Sullivan, "The MassHealth Waiver: 2009–2011 . . . and Beyond" (Boston: Massachusetts Medicaid Policy Institute and Massachusetts Health Policy Forum, February 2009) (http://masshealthpolicyforum.brandeis.edu/forums/Documents/MassHealth-waiver-2009-Issue%20Brief%20Final.pdf).

10. "State Health Facts," Kaiser Family Foundation (http://www.statehealthfacts.org/profileind.jsp?ind=198&cat=4&rgn=23).

11. Teresa A. Coughlin, Leighton Ku, and Johnny Kim, "Reforming the Medicaid Disproportionate Share Program," *Health Care Financing Review* (Winter 2000), pp. 137–57; Leighton Ku, "Limiting Abuses of Medicaid Financing: HCFA's Plan

to Regulate the Medicaid UPL" (Washington: Center on Budget and Policy Priorities, September 27, 2000); GAO, *Medicaid: HCFA Reversed Its Position and Approved Additional State Financing Schemes,* GAO-02-147 (October 2001); U.S. General Accounting Office, *Medicaid: States Use Illusory Approaches to Shift Program Costs to Federal Government,* GAO/HEHS-94-133 (1994).

12. Irene M. Wielawski, "Forging Consensus: The Path to Health Reform in Massachusetts" (Boston: Blue Cross Blue Shield of Massachusetts Foundation, July 2007), p.19.

13. John Holahan and others, "Caring for the Uninsured in Massachusetts: What Does It Cost, Who Pays, and What Would Full Coverage Add to Medical Spending?" (Boston: Blue Cross Blue Shield Foundation of Massachusetts, November 2004) (http://bluecrossmafoundation.org/sites/default/files/041116RTCCostsCaringFor UninsuredHolahan.pdf).

14. Linda Blumberg and others, "Building the Roadmap to Coverage: Policy Choices and the Cost and Coverage Implications" (June 2005) (http://bluecrossma foundation.org/sites/default/files/050621RTCPolicyChoicesBlumberg.pdf).

15. MassAct, "About MassAct" (2011) (www.massact.org/about.asp).

16. Brian Mooney, "Romney and Health Care: In the Thick of History," *Boston Globe,* May 30, 2011.

17. Michael Doonan and Katharine Tull, "Health Care Reform in Massachusetts: Implementation of Coverage Expansions and a Health Insurance Mandate," *Milbank Quarterly* (2010) (www.milbank.org/publications/the-milbank-quarterly/ search-archives/article/3475/health-care-reform-in-massachusetts-implementation-of-coverage-expansions-and-a-health-insurance-mandate?back=/issue/2010/1).

18. Mooney, "Romney and Health Care."

19. Office of Governor Deval Patrick, "Governor Patrick Announces $21.2 Billion Medicaid Waiver Agreement," press release, September 30, 2008 (www.mass.gov/ governor/pressoffice/pressreleases/2008/medicade-waiver.html).

20. Robert Seifert and Andrew Cohen. "Re-Forming Reform: What the Patient Protection and Affordable Care Act Means for Massachusetts (Boston: Blue Cross Blue Shield of Massachusetts Foundation, June 21, 2010) (http://bluecrossmafoundation. org/sites/default/files/062110NHRReportFINAL.pdf).

21. Commonwealth Health Insurance Connector Authority, "Affordability Information Sheet" (2010).

22. Massachusetts Department of Revenue, "Individual Mandate: 2008 Preliminary Data Analysis" (Boston, 2009) (http://archives.lib.state.ma.us/handle/2452/46781).

23. Massachusetts Taxpayers Foundation, "Massachusetts Health Reform: The Myth of Uncontrolled Costs."

24. Long and Stockley, "Sustaining Health Reform in a Recession"; Long and Stockley, *Health Insurance Reform in Massachusetts.*

25. Jonathan Gruber, "Evidence on Affordability from Consumer Expenditures and Employee Enrollment in Employer-Sponsored Health Insurance," Massachusetts Institute of Technology, March 2007 (http://econ-www.mit.edu/files/128).

26. Greater Boston Interfaith Organization, "Mandating Health Insurance: What Is Truly Affordable for Massachusetts Families?" (Boston, 2007).

27. Special Commission on the Health Care Payment System, "Recommendations of the Special Commission on the Health Care Payment System," July 2009 (http://www.mass.gov/chia/docs/pc/final-report/final-report.pdf).

28. Karen Davis, Cathy Schoen, and Kristof Stremikis, "Mirror, Mirror on the Wall: How the Performance of the U.S. Health Care System Compares Internationally, 2010 Update," Commonwealth Fund, June 23, 2010 (http://mobile.commonwealthfund.org/Publications/Fund-Reports/2010/Jun/Mirror-Mirror-Update.aspx).

29. Alan Raymond, "Massachusetts Health Reform: A Five-Year Progress Report," Blue Cross Blue Shield of Massachusetts Foundation (Boston, November 2011) (http://bluecrossmafoundation.org/sites/default/files/Health%20Reform%20Implementation%20Massachusetts%20Health%20Reform%205%20Year%20Progress%20Report.pdf).

30. McDonough, "The Third Wave of Massachusetts Health Care Access Reform."

31. See NCQA, "NCQA's: Health Insurance Plan Rankings: 2010–2011" (www.ncqa.org/Portals/0/Health%20Plan%20Rankings/2011/HPR2011_Summary_Report_Private_10.13.pdf).

32. EOHHS Virtual Gateway: Health Insurance and Health Assistance Programs (May 2013) (www.mass.gov/eohhs/gov/commissions-and-initiatives/vg/virtual-gateway.html).

CHAPTER 9

1. David Blumenthal and James A. Morone, *The Heart of Power: Health and Politics in the Oval Office* (University of California Press, 2010).

2. Stuart Altman and David Shactman, *Power Politics and Universal Health Care* (Amherst, N.Y.: Prometheus Books, 2011).

3. Haynes Johnson and David Broder, *The System: The American Way of Politics at the Breaking Point* (Boston: Little, Brown & Company, 1997); Altman and Shactman, *Power Politics and Universal Health Care.*

4. Center for Science in the Public Interest, "Health Reform to Deliver Calorie Counts to Chain Restaurant Menus Nationwide." March 21, 2010 (www.cspinet.org/new/201003211.html).

5. "Judge Won't Stop Abortion Insurance Law," *Boston Globe,* September 30, 2011.

6. "Anti-Abortion Groups Push for Heartbeat Bill in 50 States," *Medical Daily,* October 12, 2011 (www.medicaldaily.com/news/20111012/7387/abortion-bill-50-states-heartbeat-movement-michele-bachmann.htm).

7. Benjamin D. Sommers and others, "The Affordable Care Act Has Led to Significant Gains in Health Insurance and Access to Care for Young Adults," *Health Affairs* 31, no. 12 (December 2012) (http://content.healthaffairs.org/content/early/2012/12/13/hlthaff.2012.0552).

8. Michael T. Doonan and Katharine R. Tull, "Health Care Reform in Massachusetts: Implementation of Coverage Expansions and a Health Insurance Mandate," *Milbank Quarterly* 88, no. 1 (2010), pp. 54–80 (http://www.milbank.org/publications/the-milbank-quarterly/search-archives/article/3475/health-care-reform-in-massachusetts-implementation-of-coverage-expansions-and-a-health-insurance-mandate?back=/issue/2010/1).

9. Linda Blumberg and others, "Building the Roadmap to Coverage: Policy Choices and the Cost and Coverage Implications" (Boston: Blue Cross Blue Shield of Massachusetts Foundation, June 2005) (http://bluecrossmafoundation.org/sites/default/files/050621RTCPolicyChoicesBlumberg.pdf).

10. Abby Goodnough, "Next Challenge for the Health Law: Getting the Public to Buy In," *New York Times*, December 19, 2012 (www.nytimes.com/2012/12/20/us/officials-confront-skepticism-over-health-law.html?_r=1&).

11. Sarah Kliff, "Millions Will Qualify for New Options under the Health Care Law. Most Have No Idea," *Washington Post*, November 21, 2012 (www.washingtonpost.com/blogs/wonkblog/wp/2012/11/21/millions-will-qualify-for-new-options-under-the-health-care-law-the-vast-majority-have-no-idea/).

12. For a detailed discussion of all the elements of the ACA, see John McDonough, *Inside National Health Care Reform* (University of California Press, 2011).

13. The legislation says 133 percent of the FPL, but this is on top of a 5 percent income disregard.

14. Kaiser Family Foundation, "Quick Take: Who Benefits from the ACA Medicaid Expansion," June 14, 2012 (www.kff.org/medicaid/quicktake_aca_medicaid.cfm).

15. *National Federation of Independent Businesses* v. *Sebelius*, Sup. Ct. Dkt. No. 11-393 (U.S. 6/28/12).

16. Jordan Weissmann "Hey, Rick Perry, It'd Be Dirt-Cheap to Give More Poor Texans Health Care," *The Atlantic*, November 26, 2012 (www.theatlantic.com/business/archive/2012/11/hey-rick-perry-itd-be-dirt-cheap-to-give-more-poor-texans-health-care/265598/).

17. John Holahan and others, "The Cost and Coverage Implications of the ACA Medicaid Expansion: National and State-by-State Analysis" (Washington: Kaiser Commission on Medicaid and the Uninsured, November 2012) (www.kff.org/medicaid/upload/8384.pdf).

18. N. C. Aizenman, "GOP State Leaders Fumble by Ceding Control of Health Exchanges to Federal Officials, Critics Say," *Washington Post*, December 13, 2012 (www.washingtonpost.com/national/health-science/critics-blast-gop-state-lawmakers-for-giving-control-of-insurance-exchanges-to-federal-officials/2012/12/13/a638a4f8-452d-11e2-8061-253bccfc7532_story.html?hpid=z).

19. Ibid.

20. Julie Appleby and Christopher Weaver, "After Much Scrutiny, HHS Releases Health Insurance Exchange Rules," *Kaiser Health News*, July 11, 2011 (www.kaiserhealthnews.org/Stories/2011/July/11/Health-Insurance-Exchange-Regulations-Released.aspx).

21. Sandy Praeger, "Statement at the 20th Princeton Conference: The U.S. Health Care System in Transition" (Princeton, N.J.: Council on Health Care Economics and Policy, May 23, 2013).

22. Michael Tutty and Jay Himmelstein, "Establishing the Technology Infrastructure for Health Insurance Exchanges under the Affordable Care Act: Initial Observations from the 'Early Innovator' and Advanced Implementation States" (University of Massachusetts Medical School and National Academy of Social Insurance, September 2012) (www.nasi.org/research/2012/establishing-technology-infrastructure-health-insurance-exch).

INDEX

Massachusetts health care reform, 5, 6–7, 99–114; affordability issues, 108–09; benefits, 109–11; as bipartisan effort, 13, 100; coverage rates for, 2; impetus for reform, 101–05; implementation stage, 107–08; individual mandate in, 122; lessons for national reform, 113–14; Medicaid and federal waivers, 6, 100–101, 105; national comparisons, 111–13; provisions of, 105–07; rulemaking stage, 107–08

Massachusetts Special Commission on the Health Care Payment System, 111

Massachusetts Taxpayers Association, 104

MassHealth program, 100, 101, 112

MCC (Minimum creditable coverage), 110

Medicaid: and ACA implementation, 123–25; and CHIP implementation, 43–44, 46–47; creation of, 115; eligibility, 122; expansion of, 24–25, 48, 125; and Massachusetts health care reform, 6, 100–101, 105; matching rate for, 17; premiums, 40; and welfare reform, 8

Medicaid Management Information System (MMIS), 53

Medical savings accounts (MSAs), 18, 61, 63, 66

Medicare, 9, 12, 115

Medigap policies, 73

Mental health coverage, 37, 110

Mental Health Parity Act of 1996, 91

Merck Pharmaceuticals, 19

MEWAs (Multiple employer work associations), 63

Michigan, HIPAA implementation in, 89, 90

Minimum creditable coverage (MCC), 110

Mink, Patsy, 21

Missouri, HIPAA implementation in, 89, 90

MMIS (Medicaid Management Information System), 53

Montana, CHIP implementation in, 50

MSAs. *See* Medical savings accounts

Multiple employer work associations (MEWAs), 63

Musser, Josephine, 75, 76

Nathan, Richard, 13

National Academy for State Health Policy (NASHP), 128

National Association of Insurance Commissioners (NAIC): HIPAA implementation role of, 86, 93, 95; HIPAA legislative role of, 64, 65, 66, 69; HIPAA rulemaking role of, 73, 76, 80–81

National Conference of State Legislatures (NCSL): and ACA implementation, 128; and CHIP, 24, 32, 34, 53; on CHIP implementation, 45; and HIPAA, 64, 65, 69, 74; on HIPAA implementation, 89

National Federation of Independent Business v. *Sebelius* (2012), 3

National Governors Association (NGA): and ACA implementation, 128; and CHIP, 24, 32, 34, 53; CHIP outreach efforts by, 49; on CMS's implementation of HIPAA, 89; and HIPAA, 61–62, 65

Native Americans, 40, 41

Newborns' and Mothers' Health Protection Act of 1996, 91

New Deal, 2, 8, 115

New Jersey: CHIP implementation in, 55; CHIP rulemaking in, 37

New York: children's health insurance programs in, 20; CHIP implementation in, 45–46, 49, 50; HIPAA implementation in, 92; pre-CHIP coverage for uninsured children, 17–18

New York Times on CHIP implementation, 46

Nickles, Don, 19

Nixon, Richard, 115–16

Obama, Barack: and ACA, 2, 68, 116; on bureaucracy, 12; and Massachusetts health care reform, 99; reelection of, 3–4, 42, 122; and stakeholder engagement, 15

"Obamacare." *See* Patient Protection and Affordable Care Act of 2010

Office of Management and Budget (OMB), 32, 33, 73

Otter, C. L. "Butch," 126
Outpatient services, 37
Outreach campaigns, 49, 86, 113, 122–23

Partners Health Care System, 104
Patient Protection and Affordable Care
    Act of 2010 (ACA), 115–29; and Cen-
    ter for State-Based Health Exchanges
    (proposed), 127–28; CHIP lessons
    for, 55–56; and health care exchanges,
    125–27; implementation of, 4, 84, 108,
    121–27; individual coverage man-
    date in, 60; and Medicaid, 123–25;
    opposition to, 3–4; partisan nature of
    passage, 15, 100, 122; policy process
    for, 119–21; states as laboratories for,
    118–19
Patrick, Deval, 111
Payment level rules, 40
Peer-to-peer outreach, 113, 123
Penalties: civil, 87; for HIPAA noncom-
    pliance, 68–70, 85
Pennsylvania: CHIP implementation in,
    50; pre-CHIP coverage for uninsured
    children, 17–18
Pension and Welfare Benefits Agency
    (PWBA): HIPAA implementation role
    of, 85, 86–87; HIPAA rulemaking role
    of, 71
Personal Responsibility and Work
    Opportunity Act of 1996, 36
Peterson, Paul, 9, 10
Policymaking: for ACA, 119–21; imple-
    mentation stage, 12–13; legislative
    stage, 10–11; process of, 10–13; rule-
    making stage, 11–12
Portability of insurance, 57–58, 67,
    78–79, 93. See also Health Insurance
    Portability and Accountability Act of
    1996 (HIPAA)
Praeger, Sandy, 126
Preexisting condition exclusions: and
    ACA, 121; and HIPAA, 67, 68, 70, 77,
    80, 93, 96; and individual coverage
    mandate, 60
Premiums: as cost-sharing item,
    40; guarantees, 94; and HIPAA,
    70; in Massachusetts, 114; and

Massachusetts health care reform,
    109. See also Cost sharing
Prescription drug coverage, 37, 110
Preventive care, 110
Privacy standards, 57
Procter and Gamble, 19
Publius journal, 10

Rabe, Barry G., 10
RAND study on portability in individual
    market, 78–79
Reagan, Ronald, 3, 8, 115
Rehabilitation Act of 1973, 36
Reporting requirements: for CHIP, 26,
    38; for HIPAA, 38, 82, 83; and policy
    process, 119
Republicans: and ACA, 2; and CHIP, 16,
    18, 21, 22, 27; and HIPAA, 61, 64
Residency requirements, 35
Rhode Island: CHIP implementation in,
    51, 52, 54, 55; HIPAA implementation
    in, 89, 90
Rich, Robert, 9
Risk pool, 3, 78–79, 94
Rockefeller, Jay, 22, 60
Romney, Mitt: ACA as campaign issue
    for, 3–4; and Massachusetts health
    care reform, 6, 99, 102–05, 118
"Romney Care." See Massachusetts health
    care reform
Roosevelt, Franklin D., 115
Rosen, Dean, 65, 96
Roth, William, 18, 60
Rulemaking: for CHIP, 30–42; for
    HIPAA, 71–83; Massachusetts health
    care reform, 107–08; in policymaking
    process, 11–12; states' role in, 74–75,
    76–77, 80–83; timelines for, 72–73

Safety Net Care (Massachusetts), 112
Salvo, Matt, 89
SBA (Small Business Administration), 128
Screening for CHIP, 38–39. See also
    Eligibility
Section 1115 waivers, 101
Self-employed, 66
Senate: and ACA, 2; and CHIP, 22; and
    HIPAA, 59–62